"Living Lean is not just a 'diet book', it is a lifestyle guide. I thank John Farley for having the courage to speak about how health, weight and the power of the mind are interconnected."
— **Shary Wagreich, Chiropractor, NYC**

"I would not hesitate to recommend you."
— **David Rockefeller**

"I have lost pounds and inches, plus I feel so much better for having used your program, thank you!"
— **Gemma Denmark, Actress, NYC**

"For the first time in years you wake up in the morning thrilled to start your day. After working with John Farley, you can't wait to get through the door, out into the world, try out life with this new idea, this new tool, this new skill. You are <u>ready</u>."
— **Kristin Rudrüd, Actress,**
Fargo & Pleasantville

Living Lean!

Living Lean!

How to Lose Up to 5 lbs. Each Week
Permanently and Naturally

John J. Farley, MA

The Optimal Performance Institute
Sunnyvale, California

Second Edition
ISBN 0-9674252-0-4
Library of Congress Catalog Card Number: 99-66654

Published by   The Optimal Performance Institute
                      520 S. Murphy Ave., Suite 256
                      Sunnyvale, CA 94086

Printed and bound by Bang Printing, Brainerd, MN

Cover & text & illustration design by Janet Kucklinca

I have been working with John Farley since January 1989, and I am still shocked and delighted by the way he has virtually changed my life. As well as improving my health and fitness, he has devised a painless way for me to lose weight (20 pounds thus far), lose body fat, but most importantly alter my mindset.

I never did <u>any</u> exercise before John came along, and now I do something <u>every</u> day beyond the three mornings I work with John. I am healthier, happier, drink much less coffee and even less alcohol. All this has affected my ability to deal with a pressured, stressful job considerably.

I think John's non-threatening, enormously supportive and patient techniques are, in a quiet way, as effective as any I have seen. I recommend him with great pleasure and without any provisos to anyone like myself, totally non-motivated to exercise, or to even a sophisticated gymnast. One of John's great gifts is that he always has a surprise in store for you. I'm never bored and always challenged.

Sincerely,

Stephen Rubin
President & Publisher
Doubleday

Big deal that I lost 17 pounds in a month and two days!! No suffering or complaining (well, not a lot of complaining), just continuously feeling supported and encouraged by John Farley. Good health, including safe, challenging fitness workouts, satisfying, creative nutrition, and mental conditioning probably are the most self-perpetuating activities I have ever experienced. Once I began to feel better and saw results from working with John, I came to recognize his truly outstanding resourcefulness and effectiveness, notwithstanding his strength of character.

Going back to work after a month's vacation and getting the high-pitched accolades and hugs I did for the way I looked, only served to increase my commitment and motivation to keep working to achieve goals John and I had laid out at the beginning of our work together. Before that all who knew me would kid me about "Oh, another diet" or of my stomach's protrusion. Even the doormen in my building said when I started this program, "It'll last a month!" Now six weeks into the program and still going as strong as ever, they have congratulated and admired me. Success is the best revenge!

John has consistently treated me with great respect and good-naturedness, being sensitive to my idiosyncratic needs and habits. His gentility, patience, humor, caring and support have helped guide me to a much happier, confident, fulfilled life-style.

John never was pushy, just self-assured, enthusiastic, and quite positive that his total program of fitness, nutrition and mental conditioning was appropriate, effective and do-able, especially for one of my age group (40's), body type (chubby, at least), and habit history (no exercise past lifting menus, the telephone receiver for deliveries, eating anything and everything, indulging all impulses). His willingness to experiment with patience - challenging ideas and blocks I have, opened avenues of understanding and communication between us.

As a result of my association with John, a teacher, trainer, counselor, consultant and guru, who maintained a wonderfully positive attitude throughout our work together, I am a much happier person. I believe John's qualities are found only in truly exceptional people. I believe that such people deserve a great deal of respect.

John is an extraordinary, genuine, sensitive human being who I always will keep in the places in my mind and heart reserved for the particularly special, helpful, encouraging people who have been with me on my journey through life. Thanks John!!

Brian Kaplan, Ph.D.

To my wife Janet, thank you for the encouragement in all my endeavors. To my daughter Sally, my pride and joy. To my mother, for urging me to keep my health a top priority. To my karate teacher, Master Hidy Ochiai, for always demanding I put forth my best effort when I would have been content to do a little less. To those who donate and contribute their time to The Optimal Performance Institute by helping promote our important message to the world.

Contents

Introduction

I received a message from my mother today that a cousin of mine had died. He was a contemporary of my siblings, more than of mine, but we knew each other from many family get-togethers. At the age of 48 he died of a massive heart attack while on the job.

He had been working two jobs, was very overweight, and eating his dinners at nine in the evening. He was friendly and good-natured, well-meaning, and cared about his family. Despite these things he died much earlier than was necessary.

I am convinced that had I gotten him a copy of this book and insisted he read it and take the action steps suggested inside, he would have added many decades to his life. As my mother said to me before we hung up the phone, "when you have your health, you have everything" - when you have your health you can then go after all the other things that you want in life, but without your health the game of life comes to a close too quickly.

The truth is that while this book's title promises weight loss to you and anyone else who will do what is asked of them, it is also much more than that. This book holds within it keys to health, vibrancy, age reversal, and life extension. Wild claims? Not at all. Health is the optimal functioning of your bodily systems, vibrancy is having the energy and enthusiasm to go after what you want in life, age reversal, very simply, taking your heart and lungs, muscular strength, power, and flexibility and increasing their efficiency to a more youthful age. For example, an "Average" 50 year old man's cardiovascular ability is such that he can run 1.5 miles in 13:00-16:30 minutes. If that same man trains and is able to run the same distance in 9:30 minutes, he then is in the "Athletic" category for his age and is in the "Good" category for a 20-29 year old (one category above average). He has physiologically reversed the age and functioning of his heart and lungs from that of a 50 year old to that of a 20-29 year old.

Your life will be longer, and in many cases happier, when you live by the principles in this book. I encourage you, and everyone you know and care about, to make the principles and strategies presented to you here, a part of your daily life.

Know that you are in a battle. My cousin lost his battle to McDonald's®, Hershey's®, and an entire American culture that is overweight, stressed-out, aging, and killing themselves prematurely. It was too late for my cousin Douglas, but let his tragedy be a wake-up call to you to change your lifestyle, live longer, healthier and happier in the years to come.

Best Regards,

John J. Farley - June 1999 New York City

Chapter 1

The Double Movement Strategy

"At the end of the way is freedom. Till then patience…"
— Buddha

Congratulations, you are about to learn how to lose up to five pounds per week naturally, and also how to improve your health and fitness levels dramatically. This knowledge will not only help you, it will also help the important people in your life.

My name is John Farley and I want to share with you the art and science of mindbody fitness that I have worked hard to discover. It has cost me the proverbial "blood, sweat, and tears" to learn how to control my mind and body and I am learning more everyday. I want to show you how to get all the benefits of fitness with as much pleasure and as little pain as possible.

My lifestyle is so different today from 15 years ago I can hardly tell you. I used to be a young man (13 - 18) addicted to television and dairy products. I repressed my anger. I had asthma. Even on a good day I could barely run halfway around the block. I was in fair shape based on my 9th grade physical fitness test. By the time I was 21 I was a national karate champion, I could run one mile in five minutes, had six percent body fat and was in excellent condition. Since then I have studied how I could become healthier as well as fit. Fitness is the ability to perform a physical feat, for example, running a mile or lifting a weight. Health, however, is the optimal functioning of your entire body. Both are essential and you can have both if you can convince yourself that you deserve them. The information in this book has been used to help the more than 800 people who have been my clients or seminar attendees achieve fitness success, not to mention the untold tens of thousands who have heard me on radio and television. This book is designed to get you motivated to transform your mind and body. Parts may seem radically different than what you are used to, but read the whole book before you do anything.

The greatest obstacle between you and health and vitality is not your body, or wallet, or chocolate, or your job or the refrigerator. The only thing between you, and the body you want, is your mind. The beliefs about what you can and cannot do - should and should not do - limit you. Open your mind to new possibilities and new realities. The **Living Lean!** system will teach you powerful tools and strategies you can use to achieve your physical goals. I am asking you to challenge yourself to do more than you have done in the past. Let this program be the one that allows you to make the decision to achieve permanent weight control naturally.

By the time you are done reading this book I hope you have a paradigm shift, a belief change, and a new view of your physical capabilities. Because when you do you will not only lose up to five pounds per week permanently and naturally, but you will see yourself, food, exercise, and your life, differently as well. Having a different point of view will change your feelings and your actions for the better.

Amazingly, 66% of Americans are overweight, 58 million Americans are obese according to The American Council on Exercise, about 25% smoke, as many as 20% of the work force are alcoholics (according to Drs. Charlesworth and Nathan in their book *Stress Management,* the cost of alcoholism amounts to $15.6 billion annually), many abuse drugs, 40% are sedentary, and 50% of deaths of both men and women come from heart related disease. These statistics are likely to get worse in the near future, not better. Between stressful living, life-threatening diets and lack of proper exercise, Americans are losing the battle of the bulge.

We need to become healthier and more fit. The idea that the government should provide us with health care while we make ourselves sick is a concept worth changing. The number one requirement for making a change is to take 100% responsibility. Your results in anything in your life will come down to your ability to accept 100% of the responsibility in producing those results. Thousands of people are suing tobacco companies because the companies lied to them - the plaintiffs' claim. Wake up America! Government lies, corporate giants lie, and yet we expect to be pardoned from the disastrous effects caused by the habits that we indulge in. Not so. We think that we have time to change before it's too late. Yes, we do, but that time is running out. You need to change, to become better, stronger, more fit, now. The good news is the **Living Lean!** program can do it for you quickly. All you have to do is use the program.

No matter what you have tried in the past, recognize this to be a brand new moment. An opportunity to improve, to grow, to become better than you were before. You need some tools to create the results you want: 1) Knowledge; this will allow you to make decisions based on physical laws of conditioning and nutrition not on outdated theories 2) <u>Motivation;</u> something needs to inspire you to achieve what you are capable of - once it does you will be determined to take 3) <u>Consistent Action</u>; this will produce long term results for you as long as you are willing to 4) <u>Do Whatever It Takes</u>, to achieve your goals.

If you do not have the body that you want, then use your frustration to your advantage. You may have to work a little harder and be a little more disciplined than the person who can eat anything and still be lean or it may only take a slight change in your strategy and you will achieve fantastic results. Either way, you will no doubt appreciate your hard-earned body when you achieve it and you will most likely be healthier and live longer, too. Most of us rarely appreciate what we have until we lose it. My aunt, whom I love, smoked for 50 years before she was diagnosed with emphysema. She quit smoking immediately without withdrawal symptoms or any urge to smoke at all. Now she appreciates oxygen more than anything in the world. I believe that what we do not appreciate we will lose, be it our money, our children, our spouse, or our health and fitness.

My goal in this program is to inspire you to marvel at your own body. To be thrilled with your hidden physical potential and breakthrough to a level of physical well-being you have not experienced in a long time, if ever.

Some of the information you read in this book will no doubt be different from what you have thought to be true in the past. The German Philosopher Arthur Schopenhauer stated, all truth goes through three steps.

First, it is ridiculed.
Second, it is violently opposed.
Finally, it is accepted as self-evident.

This program is divided into strategies. Each one, when properly applied, will lead you to excellent health and fitness. Start slowly and at the same time challenge yourself reasonably.

For some of you 5 lbs. per week would be too fast; for others it would be just right. Many physiologists say that a person shouldn't lose more than 3 lbs. per week and a maximum of 4 lbs. However, they often forget (or never knew) that we cannot only lose fat during weight loss but also hardened fecal matter in the intestines. This substance is very detrimental to our health. It can add many pounds to our weight that is not fat, muscle, water, or even useful. Fecal matter lining the intestines will block absorption of nutrients and can lead to disease. In this program you will learn how to reduce it and at the same time reduce your weight. You will also learn to burn fat efficiently and create a fatburning biochemistry. Believe me, you won't be reading about this in Cosmo! Get ready to take charge of your health, your mind and your body - let's begin by learning...

The Double Movement Strategy
Revving up your internal engine

The purpose of this section is to share with you a simple and practical way to increase your metabolism, burn fat and calories, increase your energy dramatically, and help you lose weight. Before we get to the strategy itself, I want to share with you some of the popular theories on weight control. These theories are as relevant to bodybuilders as to someone overweight.

1. The Set Point Theory:

While still controversial, many scientists believe that the body/mind automatically sets the body's weight or fat percentage regardless of conscious efforts to change weight or fat. There appears to be a biological system preset which determines how much a person should eat and how much fat will be stored. It is thought that the hypothalamus, a prune-shaped cluster of nerves in the brain, may be responsible for controlling body fat and food intake. The body will keep the fat and weight of a person stable. It does this by adjusting certain physiological functions such as resting metabolic rate. A metaphor to represent the set point theory is that of a heating/cooling system. When the temperature of a room goes below 75 degrees the heater comes on; when the temperature goes well above 75 degrees the air conditioner comes on. Some people's set points fluctuate a couple of pounds and others' by 10 or 20 lbs. Questions being asked by researchers include, "does abnormal metabolism lead to obesity, or does obesity lead to abnormal metabolism?" Studies and my experience lead me to believe "yes", both can and do happen.

A series of experiments in 1960 noted by Drs. Katch and McArdle in, <u>Nutrition, Weight Control, and Exercise,</u> explains how the body adapts. Sedentary prisoners gained weight by increasing their food intake. As body weight and fat increased, concurrently the resting metabolic rate increased so it took an astounding 7,000 kcal (calories) per day for weight gain to continue! Other experiments have demonstrated that an obese person can have their metabolism decreased by reducing food intake to the point where 450 kcal (calories) per day produces no weight loss. The body will adapt and metabolisms adapt also.

2. Resting Metabolic Rate (RMR):

This is the amount of energy expended while resting. Your metabolic rate is directly related to the amount of oxygen consumed (remember oxygen; we will discuss it later). Lean body mass, primarily muscle, has a higher rate of oxygen consumption than fat does. This means the more muscle you have the more oxygen your body will consume and the more fat you will metabolize; however, that usually assumes you have the right metabolic enzymes. Studies have demonstrated that if a person has a low RMR they have up to four times the chance of gaining a large amount of weight as persons with higher RMR's. You will learn how to correct low RMR - resting metabolic rate - in this book.

3. Fat Cell Theory:

Research indicates that the severity of a person's weight issue may be related to the number of fat cells they have. It is believed that a person has a set number of fat cells. It is now thought that a person can not only increase the size of fat cells by storing more fat in them, but also increase the number of fat cells in some cases. The fat cell size can be decreased, but it appears that the number of new cells will remain once they are created. It seems logical to me, although I risk seeming simplistic, to suggest that whatever the body and mind can create it can also eliminate, including fat cells. This is currently considered "impossible." We will talk about the mind later on. Regardless of whether or not fat cells can be eliminated, the fat in them can be reduced. That means that you can become lean if you use the right program.

4. Fat-Metabolizing Enzymes:

Enzymes are absolutely critical to all functions in the body including fat metabolism. Lipoprotein lipase (LPL) is an enzyme responsible for clearing fatty acids from the bloodstream and depositing them into the fat cell. High levels of LPL enhance fat formation and may be one of the causes of increased hunger in obese people. There are also enzymes that burn fat. For examples, a result of cardiovascular endurance training, explains Dr. Ronald DeMeersman of Teachers College, Columbia University, is increased cytochrome enzymes, beta oxidative enzymes, and ketone oxidative enzymes. The result is increased fatty acid oxidation (fat burning).

The way to create more of these enzymes is to exercise at the right level. The fat-burning enzymes are like a union of workers. The union will only work when there is enough oxygen at the site (muscle, blood, cells). Without enough oxygen they go on strike and you end up out of breath - maybe even with a side pain. The key then is to give your "union" enough oxygen when you workout. That means not exercising too hard, but intensely enough to cause the union of fat burning enzymes to grow. Without continual work (exercise) the union (enzymes) disappears and no products (energy from fat-burning) are created.

The Strategy

The more intense and the longer you move the large muscles of your body the more calories you will expend. However, there is more to it than that. Theoretically, if you were to exercise for eight hours straight at moderate to high intensities you would expend a pound or two in calories in one day! Not possible you say. Marathon runners do exactly this. Have you ever seen a fat marathon runner? I rest my case. Continuous movement expends a lot of energy in the form of calories. With rare exception, overweight people move less than fit people. Your number one strategy for weight loss (and fat loss) is to get your body to burn fat and expend calories efficiently. The most important word in achieving fitness, health and fat-burning efficiency is...

OXYGEN

Your body must have enough oxygen in order to burn fat. It is only when your body can consume and use oxygen efficiently that you become a "fat-burning machine" like an elite marathon runner does. I am sure the last thing on your mind is to become a marathon runner, but I use runners as an example of people who have a highly trained fat-burning biochemistry.

Dr. Otto Warburg, 1931 Nobel Prize recipient, of the Kaiser Wilhelm (Max Planck) Institute performed cell respiration studies. He found that cells would become weak, die, or mutate when denied adequate oxygen with the exception of cancerous cells which could live and develop without oxygen. Then Dr. Harry Goldblatt substantiated and expanded Warburg's findings by removing the mutated cells and putting them into live rats. The rats injected with mutated cells developed cancer.

Another scientist, Dr. Alexis Carrel, believed that if you gave cells a clean environment and proper amounts of oxygen the cells would live forever. Dr. Carrel, a Nobel Prize winner in 1912, took tissue from a chicken's heart which would normally live 11 years. Carrel kept the cells free from their own wastes and supplied them with the nutrients they needed. The cells were kept alive 32 years until an assistant forgot to change the metabolized polluted fluid. The cells died of autointoxication. Carrel believed the cells could have lived indefinitely as long as waste products were cleaned out of the cells' environment.

The bottom line is that you must have oxygen to keep every one of your 70 trillion cells alive. Deprive your cells of oxygen long enough and you will end up with: cancer, serious back pain, cramps, headaches and excess fat on your body. I am not saying oxygen deprivation is the only reason, but it is certainly an important one.

A great inspiration to anyone who wants to get in shape, and has 101 excuses not to, is Mavis Lindgren. At age 62 she felt like 70! She attended a seminar given by a doctor and he invited everyone to a jog at 6 in the morning, so Mavis decided to join in. She could not jog even one block. So she became determined to learn how to jog and get in shape. She entered her first marathon at age 70. In 1993 she finished her 65th marathon, The New York City Marathon, at the age of 86! Nike® offered her a contract to give presentations, but she had a fear of public speaking. She used running as a way to overcome her fear of speaking and did it. The next time you're thinking you're too old, or starting too late, think of Mavis: **Don't give in, - dig in!**

You may despise the thought of exercise, but believe me it is generally an acquired taste and you can acquire it and love it, really. One strategy of exercise is to exercise for 45 to 90 minutes at a time. This can produce very good results. Our strategy is called double movement and it involves exercising twice per day, 4 - 7 days per week. Before you panic, stay with me; this is designed to be practical. You can do this, you can put it into your schedule and your lifestyle. The exercise you do is either powerwalking and/or jogging. If you enjoy jogging, good for you, if you do not then start powerwalking. Basically, powerwalking is fast walking with the arms at a 90 degree angle pumping back and forth. Do this powerwalk, or jog, twice per day for 20 - 40 minutes each time. Does this seem like too much? If so, then walk for 10 - 15 minutes each time and build up by 5 minutes each week. The key to making this work, and loving it, is to go slowly and at a comfortable pace. Do this until you prove to yourself that you're not going to pass out or throw up. My experience suggests that too many people try to get in shape overnight. It's not just people who have an overweight condition; it can be former or injured athletes, as well. Go slowly and get in the habit of the routine. Then, each week, start to challenge yourself by going longer or somewhat faster.

You may be thinking, "this can't be for real, I am not going to exercise twice a day - I don't want to workout even twice a week!" I am asking you to read the whole book before you do anything. Also, understand that this movement strategy is something you can do before work, while going to work, at lunch, coming from work, after work or before dinner.

The Science Behind This Strategy: The reason this strategy works is because you boost your metabolic rate during the first workout. As your metabolism drops back to the pre-exercise level, you exercise again to bring it back up. Here is your Fat Burning Secret: Most people think that it only matters how many calories they burn while they exercise. Actually, it matters how high your metabolism is the other 23 hours during the day. I would rather burn an extra 4 or 10 calories every hour all day than an extra 40 calories during a high intensity exercise session - and so would you. The calories you expend during the rest of the day will be largely fat, because you will be consuming more oxygen and oxygen burns fat. Give yourself at least four (4) hours in between exercise sessions. Give your body time to regain energy and in the meantime take advantage of your increased metabolism.

Here is a metaphor to help you visualize this strategy and the science behind it. Imagine two bonfires. One is large with flames going ten to twelve feet in the air. This fire is hot and intense, you can feel the heat energy. The second bonfire is more like a little campfire. You could roast a couple of marshmallows on it and that's about it. The fire represents your body's metabolism.

The small fire is kept burning by sticks and small, thin logs - these represent meals. When you put a big log on the small fire it doesn't help the fire burn, but instead the log crushes the fire and nearly puts it out. When you put the same big log on the large bonfire it burns well and is used for fuel.

This simple metaphor is how to think about the metabolisms of the lean person and the overfat person. The lean person who has trained muscles, trained enzymes, and a trained metabolism is able to burn off the meal whether it is steak, ice cream, pasta, tofu, or fruit juice. This person has a metabolism like a large, intensely hot bonfire.

The overfat person, the person with more body fat than desirable, not just a heavy person, has a metabolism like the small camp-fire. When you put that log (meal) into the fire (body metabolism) it doesn't matter very much if it is birch, oak, pine, or maple: it doesn't burn very well. The same is true for the untrained muscles, untrained enzymes, and untrained metabolism. The meal that is put in will be stored as fat if it is too large - even if it is a meal of salad.

There is a way to counter this however. The answer is to eat smaller more frequent meals/foods and make them very healthy and easily digestible. Training your metabolism and your enzymes will also teach your body to be a roaring bon fire and allow you to consume more food than ever before, without gaining fat.

It is a known fact that athletes' diets are not different in composition than the average American's - sad, but true. The one difference is that athletes eat more food and consume more calories. Think about that. They eat the same makeup of fats, carbohydrates and proteins, but the athletes consume more calories than the average person and are leaner in most cases.

Your Exercise Prescription:

I want to give you a very special method for designing your powerwalking, jogging or running program so that it is enjoyable and changes your body chemistry such that you will burn fat efficiently. I learned about the method through Dr. Philip Maffetone. He helped train Stu Mittleman. Mittleman set out to break a world record. He ran 1,000 miles in eleven days and nineteen hours! He averaged 84 miles per day and slept about 3 hours per day. He was able to produce results way beyond what most people in our society deem possible.

I want to share with you how Stu accomplished his goals and how his method will train you to burn fat and maximize your energy. Stu Mittleman graduated from the same program as myself at Teachers College, Columbia University and I had an opportunity to talk with him privately about health and fitness one day in New York City. I even sent one of my original clients to see him for some advanced fitness testing. For years, when I was personally training clients, I used the method for producing successful fitness results.

Most people exercise and perform their daily activities anaerobically (without oxygen). You, instead, want to start exercising and living aerobically (with oxygen). Anaerobic means your body is utilizing blood sugar - glucose and very little if any fat. Aerobic means you are burning a large percentage of fat and a small percentage of glucose. Some signs of anaerobic exercise and anaerobic living include: fatigue, low blood sugar patterns, recurrent exercise injuries, depression and anxiety, fat metabolism problems, premenstrual syndrome, or circulation problems and stiff joints.

To train aerobically do the following: 1) Warm up for 12 - 15 minutes. This means walk slowly or jog slowly or do whatever your aerobic exercise is going to be at a slow and easy pace in order to warm up. 2) exercise at your target heart rate for 10 - 15 minutes, 3) cool down for 10 - 15 minutes. If you start your exercise too fast and bring your heart rate up too quickly your body will not be able to move from aerobic to anaerobic back to aerobic metabolism. Instead it will stay in a high anaerobic state until you finish your exercise.

This typically results in soreness, fatigue, even dizziness. One trainer I knew would routinely cause his clients to throw up in the gym (I'm serious) because he trained them so intensely, that is, anaerobically. Unless you're trying to be a world champion, throwing up is not necessary or beneficial.

You burn mostly fat before you start exercising; therefore, you are in an aerobic state. Sleeping is very aerobic! The problem is the number of calories being burned is low even though the percentage of fat burned is high. Low calories burned means sleeping will never work for weight loss especially if your resting metabolic rate is low to begin with.

Your aim is to train your biochemistry to be aerobic while you are exercising. Preferably, for weight loss you would want to exercise for 30 - 60 minutes once per day or ideally, exercise twice per day for 30 - 45 minutes as described earlier.

Now for the art and science of the system: Figure out your target heart rate zone and then we will look at another simple and highly effective way to gauge your intensity.

180 - your age = your target heart rate (the approximate rate at which you can exercise before going anaerobic).

If you are recovering from a major illness or are on medication, subtract an additional 10 points.

If you have not exercised before, or have an injury or are gearing down in your training, or if you often get colds, or flu, or have allergies, subtract 5 points.

If you have been exercising for more than two years without any problems, while making progress in competition without injury, add 5 points.

Your Personalized Cardiovascular - Fat Burning Method:

Use the Borg Scale of perceived exertion. It is subjective and will teach you how to gauge what is happening inside your body by how intense the exertion feels.

The scale goes from 0 - 10 (see page 18). When you start

your workout, you want to feel the exertion level rise from 0 - 3 over the course of 10 - 15 minutes. Then feel as though the intensity is between a 3 - 4 on the scale for 10 - 15 minutes. Then cool down slowly allowing the blood to go back to the heart to be oxygenated instead of pooling in the muscles and increasing the toxicity in the bloodstream due to increased lactic acid and metabolites. These are exercise by-products that stop muscular contractions eventually.

To increase your cardiovascular endurance and the intensity at which you can exercise and still burn a high percentage of fat, you increase the intensity of the exercise to 4 - 5 RPE (Rate of Perceived Exertion) for one or more minutes at a time. This is the nuts and bolts of how to burn fat systematized for you. When you do this it may seem too easy; however, when you include the intensities of 4 - 5, it will become very effective for you.

The common method of identifying your target heart rate involves taking 220 - your age and multiplying it x 65-85% (this is one method). The method I am giving you here works better. Combined with the RPE scale it will work fantastically for you.

Example: 45 year old person just starting an exercise program:

1. Power walks 20 minutes twice per day.
2. Spends 80% of her time (16 minutes) at a level 3 (moderate intensity) starts slow and increases the intensity over the 16 minutes until she is at level 3.
3. Spends 15% of her time (3 minutes) at a level 4 (somewhat hard intensity)
4. Spends 5% of her time (1 minute) at a level 5 (hard intensity) exercise:
5. Cools-down for 5 minutes by walking slowly

RATE OF PERCEIVED EXERTION
(REVISED)

0
.5   **very, very light**
1.5   **very light**
2   **light (weak)**
3   **moderate**
4   **somewhat hard**
5   **heavy**
6
7   **very heavy**
8
9
10   **very, very heavy**
           (almost max.)

Choose a number that corresponds to how intense the exertion feels. This takes practice and sensitivity to how you *feel cardiovascularly*, not how you think you should feel.

What this means is that just by revving up your internal engine - your bonfire-like metabolism - you will lose weight and become more fit. Following the plan in this program, you will become tremendously healthy as well, something many athletes are not, no matter how fit they may look. From now on when you read the word "exercise" think of stoking your internal bonfire. Your bonfire (metabolism) is one key to leanness and energy.

Well-known authority Dr. Leonard Epstein has shown that people who exercise five days per week lose twice as much weight as those who exercise three days per week. Dr. Ronald DeMeersman of Columbia University's Applied Physiology Department has reported exercising four times per week doubles fat loss over twice per week. Epstein reports once - a - week exercising has no effect on weight loss, no matter how long the session. Exercise demands more nutrients, vitamins, minerals and enzymes - you MUST get the proper amounts or your exercise efforts could be wasted.

Let me say that you can not be fit without exercise. You also cannot be optimally healthy without exercise. I once coached a woman 75 lbs. overweight. She was a heavy smoker, slept very little, and constantly ate junk food. She never even owned a pair of sneakers before she met me, let alone worked-out. She had muscle cramps throughout the day and night, knee trouble and could barely walk down a flight of stairs, and often had a sore throat from smoking. She told me that although she was not fit she was basically healthy. Health does not mean you are not sick - it means optimal functioning of your body and mind. She was the furthest thing from basic health. She was a walking time-bomb.

Studies show you can look forward to these general benefits with consistent exercise:
* More efficient heart and lungs
* More stamina
* More energy!
* You will start to like and respect yourself more
* You will tend to be positive about yourself and your life
* You'll be stronger and be able to do more work with less effort
* Done properly, exercise can prevent and even reverse

osteoporosis (while calcium is important for strong bones, resistance exercises can slow or reverse bone loss. See <u>Exercise Physiology</u> by McArdle, Katch and Katch).
* Reduce anxiety and stress
* You will tend to sleep better
* Your sex life will likely improve (maybe that's why Clinton jogs! I couldn't resist.)
* You will look and feel better
* Your concentration level will tend to increase

An October 4, 1995 article in the New York Times written by Jane Brody had this to say about the benefits of exercise:
* "Regular physical activity comes closer to being a fountain of youth than anything modern medicine can offer."
* "Physical activity can halve the risk of developing heart disease or suffering a stroke. Exercise helps reduce the risk of these vascular diseases by lowering blood pressure, raising the level of protective H.D.L (high density lipoprotein) cholesterol, reducing the risk of developing blood clots and diabetes and countering weight gain."
* "Exercise lowers the risk of developing colon cancer."
* "At any age exercise is begun, it can increase the density of bones and reduce the risk of fractures."
* "Physical activity increases the sensitivity of cells to insulin, which, in turn, lowers blood sugar and the need for insulin."
* "... exercise helps people lose fat and gain muscle."
* "Exercise increases the circulation of the immune cells that fight infections and tumors."
* "Studies suggest that regular moderate exercise combined with stretching can reduce arthritic pain and the need for medication."
* "Exercise has long been known to help people overcome clinical depression ...."
* States that gastrointestinal bleeding risk is decreased with exercise.
* Memory is improved by exercise which fosters clearer thinking and faster reaction time.

* " A study by researchers at Stanford and Emory Universities showed that in older adults who were initially sedentary, regular exercise, like brisk walking, improved sleep quality and shortened the time it took to fall asleep."

The number one (1) reason for not exercising is "no time." Decide right now when you will be able to move twice during your day for 15 - 30 minutes at a time. I have heard all the excuses and the legitimate reasons why this is impossible - I am sure it is impossible for you too. Decide now that a "miracle" is going to happen in your life and you will somehow find a little extra time for yourself. Find time to be healthy or you must make time to be sick.

There is never enough time to do everything, but there is always enough time to do the important things. Time management is really priority management. Priorities come down to values. You may not value exercise, but do you value feeling good? I personally get recommitted to my health and fitness program anytime I feel ill. I also become enthusiastic after I have a great work-out or have helped a client or friend to have one. You must identify your values in order to prioritize your activities each day. If you want to know what your real values are, just write down what you spend your money and your time on. Take a moment and write down everything you do and buy for one day or one week. If what you write down does not seem to represent what you say your values are, consider re-eVALU(E)-ating your priorities in life. Remember that virtually everything in life depends on you having your health and most experiences in life are enhanced by feeling fit as well.

It is very rare for me to find anyone who does not feel better physically, emotionally, and mentally from a program of regular exercise and movement. Keep in mind: You want to walk or jog in excellent sneakers. No shoes or old sneakers, they will hurt your feet and turn you off to the experience. Wear appropriate clothes - loose or comfortable. Next, do not try to do two things at once. I am telling you - this is one of the biggest secrets to success and failure in weight loss. Those who read company reports, magazines, or do anything other than listen to music while exercising rarely get in shape. Why? Because they become more involved in the reading than the exercise and their heart rate drops, therefore, they expend fewer calories. They also move as few muscles as possible while reading and it is in the muscles where the calories get burned. I can hear you saying, " no, no, not with me - I can do both, really!" Sorry; could you play a competitive sport and read a company report, or a novel or a magazine and expect to play well? No. Become curious about the exercise process and feel your body. Music is the exception because it will cause your body to move in rhythm and sometimes more intensely. Plus, the movement often becomes associated with the music so that you actually enjoy the workout almost immediately. Aerobics classes play music; they don't hand out books.

STRETCHING AND WEIGHT TRAINING

Stretching is very important and, for most people, is an acquired taste. I personally really enjoy stretching. You don't have to think, only relax and focus. Like with virtually every part of exercise, most people go too hard when stretching - GO GENTLY- and gradually increase the intensity. It should feel like a light pulling. Included in this book is a chart of some of my favorite stretches. Hold each stretch for at least 20 seconds; one or two minutes is better. If you can not hold it that long you are simply going too intensely, too fast. Flexibility training (stretching) will release muscular tension and keep your body supple. In this regard stretching reverses aging because with age typically comes stiffness and less range of motion. You can change that with daily stretching.

Weight training is excellent for fitness. However, since our goal in this program is limited to weight loss I will not go into weight training too deeply. Rather, what you need to know is that developing your muscles will raise your metabolism, make your muscles stronger and allow you to replace fat with muscle (one cannot change into the other because they are different tissues like your arm can not turn into your leg). For our purposes you can do the upper body, abdominal, and buttocks exercises included in this book. These exercises will make sure you are shaping your muscles properly. Do them 3x per week. They will take you less than 10 minutes. For those who want to use weights here is what to do: Choose a weight that you can lift for 18-25 repetitions. Do this with excellent form (proper biomechanics) and choose a weight that gives you a slight burning sensation in the muscle around the 12th or 18th repetition. The burn is from lactic acid, a metabolic by-product. This type of routine will work your heart and lungs by increasing your oxygen demand and heart rate. Your body will become more defined with this method because you are training your biochemistry to (slowly) learn to metabolize more fat at higher intensities. Get excellent training for this - invest $50 - $150 or more for the best weight training coaching you can get, it will be worth it in results and save you from injury, I promise. While some distance runners look tired and worn out as they enter their 60's and beyond, body builders often look incredibly youthful and strong. I want to encourage you to workout aerobically and with weights to augment your fat loss results.

The reason most people do not see results when they exercise is, in my opinion, that they exercise too hard in the beginning and become injured or turned off to the experience and quit. The other reason is that they go too lightly, thus not overloading their bodies enough, and therefore, their heart, lungs, muscles and fat deposits do not change. I hope that whether you decide to exercise for vanity or for health that you take action today to put exercise into your life. Decide to make exercise using the double movement strategy part of your life. Let's go on to the next strategy.

Now for the best kept secret in nutrition, it is ...

Chapter 2

The Raw Food Strategy

"Life is a series of awakenings"
— Sivananda

As Americans we are fat. Two out of three are overweight. Dr. William Dietz of the Centers for Disease Control announced on NBC's Today show July 1999, "it is safe to say that obesity in America is epidemic." The fat-free frenzy has not helped. Our physical size and body fat percentage keep going up. What are the reasons? Commonly we are told: not enough exercise and eating too much. Not long ago the New York Times wrote two different articles on two separate days on the subjects of food and fat. One stated that restaurants were giving customers in New York City nearly twice the amount of a "regular" portion of food. This of course was to blame for the overweight of so many New Yorkers because they felt obligated to eat all of the food since they were paying for it. Another article stated that pasta was to blame for fatness because many people are insulin insensitive.

Insulin insensitive means that glucose (blood sugar) will not be metabolized properly and it eventually will be stored as fat. The marathon runner who eats a bowl of pasta will have insulin sensitive cells. The pasta will be converted to glucose (blood sugar) and used for energy. The person who has too much fat on their body may be insulin insensitive. This will cause the muscle cells to ineffectively use glucose. The glucose (carbohydrate) goes into the bloodstream and can't get into the muscle cell. Instead, the body will have many fat cells to absorb the glucose and turn it into fat. Insulin will normally cause the glucose to be driven into the muscle cells. When you are insensitive or resistant to the insulin the glucose looks for the another type of cell to enter - fat cells. The glucose is transformed into fatty acids and stored as fat. That's the basics of it.

Since exercise makes the body more sensitive to insulin, the sedentary person is less sensitive to insulin. Those who are overweight are often insulin insensitive. This means that fat is stored more easily than in the trained person. It has been suggested by some "experts" that juicing, having vegetable or fruit juices made with a juicer, and consumed is bad and fattening for you. This is not true: here's their position. They say that the fiber in the fruit and the vegetables allows the carbohydrate to be broken down slowly and released slowly as glucose into the bloodstream. Therefore, you won't have a rapid increase in your insulin levels which will drive the glucose into the muscle or fat cells. I agree that this could be a problem for some people, but there are two things to consider here: One is health and the other is weight loss. For health reasons juicing is one of the best things you can do for yourself. It supplies a large amount of vitamins, minerals, enzymes and bioflavonoids to the cells. To think that you will get enough of these things by eating cooked foods is a bit foolish. The second part is weight loss concerns. Since the hormone glucagon does the opposite of insulin within the body (it's main job is to release stored carbohydrates in the form of glucose from the liver) it might be a good idea to increase the glucagon levels so that insulin won't be overproduced. Insulin drives blood sugar levels down and glucagon drives them up. After you eat a high carbohydrate meal you, very often, get sleepy.

Here is the easy solution: have some vegetable protein powder mixed in with your juices. If you object, then have your juices with a meal that is high in fiber and has protein, like beans and rice or vegetable stir fry and tofu. This will even out your blood sugar and prevent insulin from having your glucose transform into fat and become stored in your adipose (fat) tissue.

To reverse the condition of insulin insensitivity you will need to exercise. Yes, exercise will actually change your biochemistry to become more sensitive to insulin. This in turn, will ultimately allow your body to force glucose into muscle cells to be burned as energy instead of being stored as fat. The best exercise for this is moderate-intensity aerobic (with oxygen) exercise (i.e. power-walking/jogging, biking, in-line skating, and others). One last thing on exercise - although it is not technically scientific, - you should expect to be perspiring after 10 - 15 minutes of the exercise. If not, increase your intensity gradually by going faster or making bigger arm/leg movements. If you still aren't perspiring, breathe deeper. Oxygen creates heat.

I Bet You Are Starving!

I don't mean that you are hungry. I am talking about being malnourished. Scientists are well aware that a person can be well-fed and malnourished at the same time. Consuming calories has very little to do with being well-nourished. You must take in enough vitamins, minerals, and enzymes in order to be nourished properly. Many studies within the last decade have shown that most people are deficient in several vitamins and minerals. Calories without enough vitamins, minerals and enzymes will simply lead to overweight, fatigue and disease. There are many weight-loss groups out there that teach people to weigh their food, to weigh themselves, to count calories, calculate protein, carbohydrate, and fat intake, and drink 64 oz. of water everyday. Forget it. I have never met a physically or psychologically fit person who does this! Only those with weight concerns do. The whole ritual of weighing and measuring becomes an obsession. You can eat a loaf of white bread and get 1,500-1,700 calories, but still manage to miss out on all the vitamins, minerals and enzymes. Allow your body to have access to the nutrients it needs and you will be healthier and more fit. I have counseled women who have been through programs that require weighing and measuring every minute of the day and they come to me because they just can't lose that last five pounds and they are afraid to eat any less food. It is not the calories they should be concerned about, rather it is the nutritional value of the food.

DEAD FOOD - DEAD BODY

I am going to tell you something that perhaps no one has told you before. You are not what you eat, but you are what your cells absorb and use. The vast majority of the people that are in this country and in industrialized nations around the world eat dead food, not live food. Dead food is one major cause of chronic disease and overweight for people in the world. It is the one type of food virtually everyone eats and it is the underlying cause of degenerative disease for most people. Minimizing or eliminating cooked food will unleash your body's healing potential by freeing up energy and providing nutrients.

Enzymes are Life!

You may have been taught in school, as I was, that enzymes

are protein molecules. There is more to an enzyme than that, let me show you. An enzyme is like a battery. A battery has "juice" in it and can "energize" a radio, for example. When the current, force, or juice is used up, the battery can no longer energize the radio. The physical battery is still there. You cannot tell if it is full of juice or not by looking at it. The battery looks the same, full of energy or not, but without energy, it is useless.

Like the battery an enzyme has "juice" or "force", it is in fact living. Enzymes are involved in every process in the human body, including fat metabolism and energy production. When enzymes are heated past approximately 126 degrees Fahrenheit, they are completely destroyed (for more on this see Enzyme Nutrition by Dr. Edward Howell, Avery Publishing Group, 1985). The enzyme may look like it did before the heat, but like the battery after it is used up it is useless, dead. Without enzymes life does not exist. Enzymes digest all of our food for us. When we eat foods that have not been heated nor spoiled the enzymes are alive. These live foods have the enzymes in them to break-down the food and help metabolize it. Every time you eat a processed or cooked food lacking in live enzymes your body's organs and tissues must secrete the necessary enzymes to digest the food. Enzymes are critically important to your health, energy, and weight. Here is what you need to know about enzymes and raw food:

1. Enzymes are involved with every process in your body.

2. Raw food (not processed and not cooked over 126 degrees F) contains enzymes that predigest the raw food as we eat it (i.e. a banana sitting out too long becomes overly ripe and its enzymes start to digest it).

3. Cooked and processed foods have no live enzymes. It's dead food. Your body must draw enzymes from your organs and tissues to digest the food. Some experts suggest eighty-five percent of the original nutrients are either destroyed or made unavailable. This takes away your energy. Michael T. Murray, N.D. states that digestion is the body process that utilizes the greatest amount of energy.

4. Your body now has a deficiency in nutrients. This deficiency of nutrients causes your body to experience cravings (food allergies are another cause).

Those cravings cause you to feel hungry, when in actuality your body really needs nutrients. As you eat more cooked and processed foods you receive 100% of the calories and very little of the nutrients. Even eating raw vegetables whole only gives as much as 35% to as little as 1% of the food value. The average person according to a 40 year nutritional veteran, Jay Kordich, receives only 10% of the food value of the foods they eat. We would have to eat 15 lbs. of vegetables every day in order to get the nutrients we need. By juicing the foods with a juice machine (not a blender) you separate the juice from the fiber. The fiber is used to facilitate the removal of waste through the colon. It is the juice trapped within the walls of the fiber that contains the nutrients. IT'S THE JUICE OF THE FIBER THAT FEEDS YOU. That has been Kordich's slogan for 40 years. Here is the one thing that I bet no one has ever told you before about digestion: YOUR BODY IS NOTHING MORE OR LESS THAN A JUICE EXTRACTOR DURING DIGESTION. Its job is to separate the juice from the fiber. When you use a juice machine to do the job, you allow the body to take a rest, conserve its energy, and get up to 92% of the food value of the food instead of 10%, on average, from eating it whole.

IT IS NOT WHAT YOU EAT THAT COUNTS, IT IS WHAT YOU ABSORB THAT MATTERS!

I had been through six and one-half years of professional physical education and exercise science education at some of the best schools in the country, as well as attending conferences and seminars and no one ever told me that! It is hard to dispute. Even mainstream media admits that everyone needs to eat more fruits and vegetables. Don't expect them (government, hospitals, drug companies, television commercials ...) to tell you what you are reading here - you must evaluate it for yourself and decide for yourself. The power to achieve health, energy, leanness, and vitality is largely contained in your daily consumption of fresh raw vegetable juice and the eating of fresh fruit, as well as seeds, beans, sprouts, and whole grains provided they are not overly heated.

COOKED FOOD CHANGES YOUR METABOLISM

The glandular secretions of the pancreas and pituitary glands will become exhausted from over-stimulation resulting from a diet of cooked food. The body becomes sluggish because of the extra activity it must perform. The thyroid also becomes exhausted, resulting in gained weight. Farmers have proven this by feeding raw potatoes to hogs so they would not get fat. When cooked potatoes were fed to the hogs they gained weight rapidly and could then be sold for more money. Eating cooked food will do the same to you!

When it comes to body fat:
THE FAT GET FATTER and THE FIT GET FITTER

It is easier to stay overweight (overfat) than to become lean. It is also easier to stay lean than it is to gain weight. You may be saying that you can easily drop weight but your problem is keeping it off. Once you make the fitness and health principles in this program part of you, and you live it, breathe it, drink it, eat it, walk it, and talk it, you will laugh at chocolate cake. You will have mastered it because you will have mastered yourself and your body and mind - it's true.

The key is to experience yourself as if you were on a journey, not a "get the goods and try to hold on to it" mentality. If you are constantly doing your best to maximize your energy, strength, endurance, flexibility, and oxygen consumption, you will never have to worry about your weight. Your weight will take care of itself.

MOST PEOPLE ARE SUBCONSCIOUSLY
PLAYING THE WEIGHT LOSS LOTTERY!

The lottery is what nearly everyone hopes to win so that they can quit work or do what they love to do, or do nothing and feel financially secure. Unfortunately, achieving something so easily is the downfall of some people. They didn't work to get the money and many squander it or spend it foolishly. Within a short amount of time they find that this "found money" is spent. What would you do if you won $200? Most would spend it. Few people would actually put it in a savings account. Even when the winnings are much more, the same mentality takes over. Even if they don't spend it, many people will develop a "try not to lose it" mentality. This mentality prevents them from learning how to create more money and keep it all circulating in the universe. The "try not to lose it" mentality is also the primary mindset of most dieters. They think, "if I can just lose 15 lbs. that would get me motivated to exercise and eat better." Sorry, it may seem logical, but I have never seen it work. If it did work then the majority of weight loss programs would not have so many long term failures (or scale neurotics; those focusing too often on the scale). You will hear me say it again throughout this book; it is your mind that determines your ultimate success or failure.

STOP PLAYING THE LOTTERY AND START THE JOURNEY

The journey I am talking about is like taking a bike ride through a wooded park. You pack a lunch, and start off on the ride. You carry a map with you for guidance and know when you want to arrive and where. You enjoy the ride as you go. Sometimes the ride may be hard and uphill, but you do it anyway. Sometimes it's easy and you can coast downhill. Others times you may come across friends during your ride and decide to stop and visit. Other times you will have to discipline yourself to stop talking and ride. Even when you get to the destination, you recognize it as a plateau. Soon you will set out on a new journey to another place, another plateau. You will have flat tires along the way, it may rain, it may be sunny, hot, cold, windy, crowded, or empty, but you love it for the challenge and the adventure that it is!

Here Is Your Weight Loss Strategy

1. Eat live, fresh fruit only, in the morning - as much as you want up until noon. Avoid coffee, milk, toast, bagels, muffins, etc. If you eat melons eat them alone. The reason is melons with other fruits tend not to digest well. If this is not a problem for you, don't worry about it. Beware that mixing these fruits could cause digestive unrest.

2. Buy digestive enzymes and take them as directed with every cooked or processed meal you eat. These enzymes ought to digest fat, protein, and carbohydrate.

3. Drink at least 12 oz. of carrot-apple juice each day. It doesn't store well so drink it soon after you make it so that the nutrients do not oxidize. If you want to add any green vegetable to the carrot-apple (i.e. spinach), that would be even better for you. Adding a variety of vegetables to your juices gives you different vitamins and minerals. The fruit and the juice will help to detoxify your body, give you maximum nutrition and food value, as well as help you eliminate toxins from within the colon. This could get you to your weight loss goals by itself, I have had many clients do it, but add the power of..

Chapter 3

The Supplemental Strategy

"If the average person took as many natural supplements in place of all the medications, alcohol, cigarettes, vaccinations, aspirins, and cough suppressants normally consumed, they would be remarkably healthier"

— John Farley

I originally studied nutrition in my undergraduate coursework. I was taught that supplements were not necessary for those who have an adequate diet. I lived my life on that principle for many years after college. I thought the selling of vitamin-mineral supplements by some of the other people in the health and fitness industry was a scam. I would have nothing to do with selling supplements. However, I did come away from my traditional education with a belief that a supplement was good insurance against a possible deficiency of nutrients. Years later, higher education has only changed a little. It took years of considering research and my own personal experiences with optimal nutrition to change my mind. I became convinced that your likelihood of having an adequate diet is not possible on the average American diet. A former company of mine proudly provided excellent nutritional products to people who could benefit from them. I decided that if I was going to encourage and even require that my clients take supplements then they might as well buy them from my company. The probability of you or me having an adequate diet is very slim. The probability of anyone having an optimal diet is even smaller, therefore, supplementation is useful if not *absolutely necessary.*

The factors that will influence your nutrient needs include: your personal genetic requirements, gender, activity level, age, health status, stress level, fitness goals, nutrient absorption ability, medications, and the food you consume. It is hard to find anyone without stress in their life - positive or negative stress. Any of these factors create a situation whereby it is nearly impossible to be nourished adequately not to mention nourished optimally. Linus Pauling, Ph.D. a chemist, physicist, mathematician, Nobel Prize recipient and nutritional researcher, has shown scientifically that Vitamin C can prevent the common cold or lessen the severity of it. Until his death, a few years ago, he remained convinced of the powers of vitamin C and supplementation. Books can be filled with supplementation research. You can read them or take Dr. Pauling's word for it. I suggest you do both. Test it out for yourself; take supplements and read up on the latest information.

A COMPLETE SUPPLEMENTATION FORMULA

You may be taking a multivitamin supplement giving you 100% of the RDA (Recommended Daily Allowance - a government standard set by scientists), but be aware that the RDA is the bare minimum and only provides enough nutrients to prevent disease with a small amount of "cushion". The RDA is set for healthy people only, not those with medical conditions. The problem is that being over-weight is a medical condition, as is high stress, constipation, high blood pressure, diabetes, and any other condition causing a deple-tion or greater usage of nutrients. Even traditional nutritionists re-port that half the country would have nutrient deficiencies if they consumed 100% of the RDA for those nutrients. The moral is that you need supplementation and you need more than 100% of the RDA.

Linus Pauling recommended taking 1,000 mg. of vitamin C every *hour* when you had a cold. The RDA is 60 mg. a *day*. Supple-mentation can make the difference for you in weight loss too. If you are deficient in chromium for example, you will not metabolize fat well. There are many nutrients that you will want to increase your intake of. The question you may still be asking is if supplementation will really help you lose weight. Dr. Michael Colgan of Rockefeller University did studies over many years and found that 8 out of 10 (80%) people using vitamin-mineral supplements properly, on his program, lost weight and kept it off for 8 years without weight gain. Here are some supplements you can begin taking. Start with 2-3 supplements at a time and add 1 or 2 each week to allow your body to accommodate the change. Here are supplements I and other pro-fessionals recommend for weight loss and lean muscle improvement:

Supplement:	Amount:	Effect:
Psyllium	As directed on label	Fiber; bowel movement
Kelp	As directed on label	Balanced minerals with iodine; aids weight loss
Lecithin	As directed on label	Breaks down & emulsifies fat
Spirulina	As directed on label	Excellent source of usable protein; contains nutrients; stabilize blood sugar

Vitamin. C	3,000 - 6,000mg/day	Normal Glandular function
L-Carnitine	As directed on label	Increase endurance, increase metabolism.
L- Phenylalanine	As directed on label	Shuts hunger center down
L- Arginine	500 mg each	Not for children or diabetics
L- Ornithine	As directed on label	Take to avoid imbalance
L- Lysine	As directed on label	The above amino acids with this one decrease body fat
B Complex with B12 and B6	50 mg. 3x per day	Removes excess water
Vitamin E	400 IU (internat. units)	Important for fat metabolism.
Chromium Picolinate	200 mcg	Regulates insulin & cravings
Multi-Vitamin-Min.	As directed on label	Eliminates deficiencies
Pycnogenol	90 mg	lowers the risk of heart disease. Over 100 other benefits.
Coenzyme Q 10	Up to 100 mg	Brings a slow metabolism back to normal to enhance fat burning. Many benefits.

When you purchase your supplements, avoid inexpensive products. If they are cheap, they may have little nutritional value and plenty of fillers. The key to supplements is taking them regularly. Many people buy supplements and only take them once in a while or when they have a cold. Take them daily and vary the amounts and types every month or two. This will keep your body from becoming stale. Just like when you do the same exercises over and over with no change, your body does not improve and can actually become less fit. Now let's learn a great secret for achieving health and weight loss, it is...

Chapter 4

Fasting for Fat Loss Strategy

"We do not see things as <u>they</u> are. We see them as <u>we</u> are"
— The Talmud

As mentioned before, your success will be ultimately determined by your mindset. We will cover mindset more in the later part of this special book. For now, understand that your thoughts determine your feelings and your emotions will drive your behaviors. The failure state of mind is typical of the person who says, "I just won't eat, then I'll lose weight." This person is thinking short-term and out of deprivation. Fasting and modified fasting, as I will share with you here, is a different mindset. It is the mindset of healing, recovery, and rejuvenation. This mindset is the winning mindset; use it.

Myth #1: "If I don't eat I'll get ill, weak and tired, won't I?"

Truth #1: Less food to digest will cause your body to have more energy and strength.

Myth #2: "Fasting will cause me to binge, won't it?"

Truth #2: It is possible, but more likely to happen if you were to use a complete fast and have the wrong mindset. What I am suggesting here is that you use a modified fast, as I will explain, and have the proper mindset. That way bingeing will be unlikely.

Myth #3: "Won't fasting put my body into a starvation mode and cause me to store fat even more than before?"

Truth #3: With regular dieting it frequently does do this causing a yo - yo dieting syndrome. Fear, anxiety and deprivation will also cause your body to slow down and prepare for starvation. That is why a modified fast, one that gives you food and nutrients, done with an attitude of excitement and joy will create fat loss.

Here is the four-day modified fast I recommend to you:

Day One: Eat fresh fruit <u>only</u> all day. Drink water periodically. Eat as much as you want!

Day Two: Eat fresh fruit, <u>only</u> for breakfast. Have carrot-apple (spinach optional) juice for lunch; then fresh fruit for lunch; Fresh fruit for dinner.

Day three: Fresh fruit for breakfast; carrot-apple juice during the morning. Carrot - apple (spinach optional) at lunch time with a raw vegetable (only) salad. Dinner; carrot - apple juice; then fresh fruit. Then, if hungry, 20 minutes later, a vegetable only salad.

Day four: Begin to eat "normally' (normally will be different for you by the time you are done with this book) and eat lightly. Avoid shocking your system with heavy foods, or your body will let you know about it by the way you feel.

You can expect to lose a few pounds with this modified fast, as well as give your body a much needed rest from intense digestive work. If for some reason you do not lose weight, relax, and continue exercising. No matter what, you will have increased energy and that means you will have more motivation to be active. Should you take any supplements while doing this fast? Yes. Take your multivitamin-mineral supplement. One of the best ones I have found is Vitamin Power's Nutra Source 100, it's excellent and will make sure you are getting the nutrients you need to stay healthy and lose weight too. I also recommend spirulina because of the high protein and nutrient content of this food source. You should know that fasting in this manner without supplements is likely to be fine as well, but as we discussed, supplementation has proven to be necessary. I recommend, as do many professionals and doctors, that you fast in this manner three days every month for your continual health and longevity.

I hope you agree with me that this modified fast is very doable. It is your MIND that will determine your success or failure over those four days. Some people do these types of fasts for 5 or 10 days for maximum health benefits. It is also a good idea to start with a one day fast, especially if you feel as if a four-day modified fast is too long for you at this point.

BONUS INFORMATION: When you are sick -fast. Give your body the rest it needs without having to expend energy needed for recovery and healing on digestion and assimilation of food. Take in more supplements and herbs than you do food. This way you will recover faster and end up being healthier. I am rarely, if ever, ill for more than one week per year, maximum. I have seen others come down with the same cold that I have gotten and be sick for 3 or 4 weeks! I have also seen people never have a sniffle until learning they have a terminal illness. The body can tolerate a lot of toxins, for a while, and then you have to pay for it.

Also, do not chew anything, like gum while you are fasting (or anytime really). Chewing triggers the digestive enzymes and secretions into the gastrointestinal tract. Without any food in your stomach for these enzymes to digest problems can occur. Fasting like this will also allow your body to metabolize your body's fat stores for energy, as well as foster the removal of waste and fecal matter from your intestines. You could lose a few pounds simply from allowing this fecal matter to be removed from your colon. That is also why whole fresh fruit and even psyllium is excellent for you to consume. The fiber will move that decaying matter out of your body.

Contra-indications to Fasting

In advanced cases of diabetes, active tuberculosis, active malignancies, mental diseases and weak hearts in older patients, fasting is not recommended. Where there is any kind of disease, do not attempt fasting without consulting your doctor and abiding by his decision on the advisability of undertaking a fast in your situation. Now let's turn our attention to an important and often overlooked subject, the ...

Chapter 5

The Body-Mind Strategy

"Flow with whatever may happen and let your mind be free: Stay centered by accepting whatever you are doing. This is the ultimate"
— *Chuang Tzu*

In 1993 I was asked to be a presenter at the mind-body fitness conference in Santa Fe, New Mexico. I was presenting with many top leaders in the field: Larry Dossey, M.D., Miron Borysenko, Ph.D., Irving Dardick, M.D., Suzy Prudden, and many others. Everyone gave fascinating information about mind - body interactions. I was at the conference to present my FireWalking Seminar, the same seminar that I demonstrated on Good Morning America Sunday where the host walked across the hot coals and described the experience as "unbelievably exhilarating!!" (The FireWalk is a seminar where you learn to overcome your fears and limiting beliefs and trigger a peak performance mental state. This state enables participants to walk barefoot over very hot coals safely). In Santa Fe, all 50 of the attendees who came to my seminar walked across the coals barefoot without injury. They all overcame the learned fear of fire, achieved the optimal state of mind to walk successfully and they completed the walk safely.

The difference between walking over the coals, or not, is mastering fear. All it takes is the ability and willingness to conquer that fear, channel it into challenge and excitement and you will walk across the hot coals and love it. It is the same with weight control. You must overcome the fear, or doubt or negative association that you feel when you think of achieving or striving for permanent leanness. Your mind will be your greatest friend or your worst enemy.

Dr. Maxwell Maltz wrote a book called Psycho-Cybernetics decades ago and it is still very popular today. Maltz said, in essence, our brain has a goal seeking mechanism in it. That goal seeking mechanism directs all of our thoughts, words, images and behaviors to match up with our self-image of ourselves. Most often our true self-image is below our conscious awareness - it is subconscious.

Your subconscious mind is very powerful. Your subconscious mind will cause you to perform behaviors your conscious mind told you not to do. For example, many people consciously decide to quit smoking; however, they often experience automatic reactions to "light up" in certain situations that trigger smoking for them. These strong desires or automatic reactions are driven subconsciously, not consciously. You may resist your subconscious desire to smoke, but the brain at a deeper level still believes that smoking is: good; sexy;

rebellious; glamorous; macho; relaxing; enjoyable....

You have not reconditioned your subconscious mind to relabel smoking. For example, as I mentioned earlier, my aunt smoked for 50 years. Then she went to the doctor because of her breathing and was told she had emphysema. My aunt quit immediately. She never had withdrawal symptoms, she never had cravings, and she will not be around others smoking. She was able, somewhat spontaneously, to recondition her brain, fast! She now associates smoking with massive pain: physical, emotional, and psychological - and no benefits at all. She associates staying away from smoking to better breathing, although now her breathing is severely impaired.

The key is to take control of the mind. Sometimes this can be done consciously by making a decision to act differently. Other times it requires outside help: therapy, hypnosis (more on this later) or a life-altering event. Freedom can be yours when you decide how you want to look and break through any fears or limiting beliefs to your success.

Eating Disorders and What To Do About Them

The following is a questionnaire adapted from an article in IDEA Today, May 1994. It was presented by Michelle Mallozzi, M.S., RD. The list is incomplete and signs may vary in intensity depending on the individual. Can you answer "yes" to these questions?

* Workouts are forced and dragged out.

* Energy is low.

* Performance does not improve.

* Body shape does not become more defined, and you still "see" body fat in the mirror, no matter how many exercises you do and how little you eat.

* Stealing food or exercise equipment becomes a problem.

* You don't want to eat in front of other people.

* You are preoccupied with thoughts of food, weight, fat calories and dieting, which relates to an obsession with exercising to change your body appearance, for example, doing countless repetitions of leg exercises to tone muscles and slim down legs, even though everyone tells you your legs are not fat.

* Guilty feelings arise about eating too much. This may lead to binge - purge behavior.

* You take diet pills to lose weight and/or use steroids to increase muscle an decrease body fat.

* You think everyone is looking at you in the gym because of your looks, or you keeping looking around at people in the gym and comparing yourself to them, wishing you had their thighs, waistline, etc.

* You experience changes in sleep patterns, feelings of being out of control, depression, anxiety, mood swings, low self-esteem.

* You feel an intense need to be accepted by others, especially by having the perfect body. You strive at all costs to have that body but never reach the point where you are happy with how you look.

* You suffer from headaches, bloating, cramps or gastrointestinal problems.

* You become very upset if someone makes a comment about your body, regardless of whether it is a compliment ("You look great") or criticism ("You need to work on your upper body a bit more to make your body look more evenly defined").

If you think you have an eating disorder, you have already taken the first step, recognition. I have had the honor over the years to assist many people in getting in shape and altering their life-styles. In my experience women, in general, have a harder time achieving health and fitness goals as a group. Some women are able to get into great shape - go to any serious health club and ask around; you will find women who have lost 100 lbs. or more and look so good you might not believe it. The challenge for most women is primarily psychological and to a certain extent physical. Even men can have as many, if not more, psychological blocks to life-style change than women. We could fill another book on why women tend to have this, but it is not necessary for our purpose here.

Kelly Brownell, Ph.D. of the University of Pennsylvania's Obesity Research Clinic, has studied the negative thought patterns of those wanting to lose weight. Brownell says overweight people tend to split their lives into two separate compartments - "on" a diet and "off" a diet, never in between. I have seen this thinking in many women; occasionally in men and more often in overweight men. Brownell also sees a second negative thinking pattern. The pattern is when dieters set unrealistic goals for themselves and feel guilty about not reaching them. This book says you can lose up to 5 lbs. each week. If you set your goal at 5 lbs. and only lose 4 lbs. you will have failed to meet your goal. If you put your goal at 1 or 2 lbs. and lose 2 or 3 you will have met your goal and probably feel successful.

The third negative thought/behavior pattern Dr. Brownell has identified is what we can call "absolute thinking." Brownell says dieters establish strict rules that are very difficult to live with. For example, "I will never eat chocolate again" "I will never stop for fries on the way home" "I will never buy a donut at work." When you fail, you tend not to forgive yourself, he says. The last thought pattern Brownell sees, is dead-end thinking. It is based on envy. Anytime you focus on what other people have or can do and feel envious or angry about it, you have slipped into this thought pattern. "She eats everything and still loses weight and I just look at fudge and gain a pound!" The only place this gets you is back to square one.

It's Your Mother's Fault!!

Some researchers and scientists have found a correlation between overweight young women and their having mothers who habitually criticize their appearance. For many people their body is the one thing they can "take control of" - so they eat. If you do that, let me give you a different "frame" to consider: *Success Is The* Best *Revenge.* Decide that being healthy, happy and fit are more important than playing childish power games, that in reality only hurt you, because no one else has to live in your body except you. Forget blaming your mother or anyone else. Take total responsibility for yourself and take action. Many researchers suggest that overeating is closely related to poor self-concept. Self-concept and self-image is what self-image psychology and psycho-cybernetics are based on. Understand that it is not "I have a good (or poor) self-concept." Instead we all have many self-concepts. You have a self-concept of yourself as a driver, a singer, a typist, an artist, a bowler, a golfer, a runner, a student, a business person, a mother, a child, a spouse or significant other and more. All of these self-concepts are different. You may say, "but John, I don't golf at all" - then your self-concept is unformed -but I am sure you have a self-image/concept of how smart you are. Most people think of themselves as smart, dumb or average. However, it was Dr. Howard Gardner of Harvard University who first put forth the concept of Multiple Intelligences. Multiple Intelligences says that you and I have at least seven different areas in which we may be considered intelligent or not, but we are not simply intelligent or unintelligent. What I am saying is that you do not have *a* poor self-concept, you may have 10 poor self-concepts! Or you may have a poor body self-concept and still believe that you are a brilliant artist, or stockbroker. The point is that you LEARNED to create everyone of those concepts and you can learn and relearn to create your "body self-concept." You do it by visualizing yourself succeeding, affirming yourself as deserving of your end result, and imagining yourself achieving those results - feeling great about those results and repeating it daily. You also acknowledge your successes and take responsibility for your defeats.

THE 7 FAT FEARS and NEGATIVE ASSOCIATIONS

I have seen "experts" in weight control state, very boldly, that psychological factors are not involved in overeating, obesity, and overweight conditions, that these are physiological conditions. I have heard other "experts" claim that you can not permanently lose weight until you have healed yourself in mind and spirit. Our work with a variety of people over the years has convinced me of the power of the mind, body and spirit (life giving principle within us). You can be thin and have mental problems, as well as physical ailments, as well as evil intentions. You can be overweight and have no overt ailments, be very well-adjusted and feel good about yourself, as well as be very compassionate and giving towards others.

If you want to transform your body and mind then you need to understand how your body-mind functions. What about motivation? Motivation is crucial to your success in weight control and we will explore motivation secrets. We will look at fear and neuro-associations to determine how and why we think and act the way we do. Fear is the great paralyzer of human action. Overwhelming fear can stop us in our tracks, literally, without allowing us to move a muscle. What we associate to things determines our actions. Let me explain. Write down what you associate to the word "exercise" _____. At my seminars I will often ask the participants to tell me what they think of when I say the word, "exercise." I get varied responses; often, "pain," "Yuk!," "boring." "intimidating," "gray paint on the wall," and sometimes "invigorating," or "challenging." I associate discipline, control, power, and secret skills to the words "martial arts" - a type of exercise. This is what we call your association to exercise. This association is not just a thought; it is in fact an entire mindbody representation. You are not just thinking "Yuk" or "exciting" or whatever word you wrote, you are feeling it! When a person has a phobia they will often experience physiological symptoms even when they imagine the trigger of the phobia (i.e. elevators, dogs, snakes, spiders). The vivid thought (although almost always subconscious) will create the physiological reaction.

You have associations to: food in general, specific foods, exercise in general, specific activities, being lean, fit, healthy, attractive and millions more. Many studies have shown that by creating or changing associations to a stimulus we can change a response. This is what Ivan Pavlov did. Pavlov was the scientist with the dogs, the bell and the meat. He waited for the dogs to get hungry, and when he gave them meat he rang a bell. After enough repetition the dogs associated, in their nervous systems, a new response to the bell. Now, when Pavlov rang the bell the dogs salivated -an unconscious activity - in anticipation of meat. You have associations that influence your ability to reach your weight management goals, as well as all of your goals in life. The question is, can you identify what they are and recondition yourself for success? Let's go through the 7 fat fears (or negative associations):

1. Fear of Facing Pain: If you use food to comfort yourself after emotional discomfort; or if you are unwilling to workout because you do not want any discomfort then this may be a negative association influencing your life-style.

2. Losing Authority/Attention: If you associate size to power, control, attention, or authority then this could be a negative association in your life.

3. Food as Reward/Entertainment: Do you associate food to parties and get-togethers, to jobs well done, to fun. Do you eat the token vegetable on your plate and reward yourself with dessert after?

4. Food as Love/Nurturing: When you experience hurtful emotions, or "negative" emotions, do you eat to feel better emotionally?

5. Fear of Intimacy/Sexuality: This fear manifests as an aversion to relationships, to sex (even with a longtime spouse), or aversion toward allowing others to get to know you. Staying large allows a physical barrier to come between you and others.

6. Fear of Loss of Identity: This is evident in your language. Are you a heavy, large, overweight, or a compulsive, overeating person? Do you refer to yourself as, "I am overweight." Do you use genetics as a reason for your situation? Is it just something about the way you are that causes your condition? Is your weight, "just the way you are?" The fear involved in this situation is: who would you be if you were not overweight? Could you imagine yourself as Ms./Mr. slim and trim? How would you relate to the other people in your life? How would they treat you if you were lean and slender - the same, different or are you unsure?

7. *Fear of Change:* Everybody seems to want things to get better, without changing. The only way things get better is through change. In a way, this fear is a general fear of the last six and other specific fears not mentioned. Something about the way you are living is comfortable for you or you would do whatever is necessary to change it.

Possibly the most empowering neuro-association to have is in the form of a belief. Our beliefs about who we are, our capabilities and about the world are really a set of neurological associations. I demonstrate this in my FireWalk seminar. The participants come to the seminar with preconceived ideas about fire, heat, and skin. About 4 1/2 hours later they are living in a different reality that says "I can walk on hot coals safely and like it!" Then they do it. Their belief affects their body and provides an immunity - it might be hard for you to believe, but we have tested it and the results are hard to deny. The same happens in the placebo effect. Scientists enjoy discounting results that are based on the placebo effect or the expectations (belief) of a person. Yet the placebo effect is a demonstration of the power of belief to change a person's biochemistry (in the case of administration of drugs vs. placebos). Giving a person an aspirin and another a sugar pill and telling him it is aspirin is common. If the headache goes away with the sugar pill it is very possible that the subject's expectation of successful relief generated an actual change in his biochemistry. The reverse happens as well. No matter how many drugs are given to someone, if they want to be in pain or even die, their mind can create it.

My karate teacher told once of an experience when he was about six years old. His master in the temple in which they lived in Japan told him that they would be going on a three day trip to see another master who was 85 and was going to die on the third day. He went on this trip and saw the master and his death. He was struck by the idea, even at that young age, that a human being could will his own death.

The mind and its beliefs are powerful. Here is a belief or association you might want to adopt: "I am perfectly imperfect." Accept the idea that you are imperfect - and that's exactly how you should be. Then work to improve, learn and grow as a person. No matter how thin or rich you are you'll never be perfect so learn to live with it. Then once you accept yourself as imperfect, tell your friends that you're not perfect, admit your mistakes, take responsibility for them, and laugh about them. Take a moment to reread this paragraph, it is important for your success and peace of mind.

When I was preparing for a national karate tournament in 1987, I was a little nervous about the competition. I knew all my friends and students were wishing me well and my mother was, as always, concerned about my safety. I was meditating the night before about the event. I was thinking about how hard I had trained and how I would perform. Then, I thought to myself: "If I lose, what's the worst that would happen?" "Some people might be disappointed." Then I thought; "but my friends will still like and respect me, and my mother will still love me and so will my family." That shift took a lot of pressure off of my mind. I went and competed in the tournament, and I won first place and third place in the two events.

IDENTIFY YOUR BLOCKS TO SUCCESS

Many people are in massive denial. If you're in big time denial you might not have even made it to this page. But even some denial could be the missing link in your permanent weight control quest. What is the real reason that stops you from achieving your fat loss /body shaping goals? I cannot answer it for you, but I can give you a simple little quiz to help you discover it for yourself. Take a deep breath and ask yourself these questions and WRITE the answers down on paper:

1. What is stopping me from achieving permanent weight control? Please answer this question to the best of your ability. Do not think all day, just start writing and let the thoughts flow. Then when you think you have answered it go to the next question.

2. What does my current life-style (that is promoting my overweight condition) do for me that's positive (or useful)? Consider this for a moment. I usually get "nothing" as an answer when I first ask this question. For example, not exercising often is a way for a person to get more business done. Eating fast food is sometimes a way to make it to a meeting on time or it is the "social" thing to do with your friends - it is therefore, a way to maintain your friendships by eating together. Every action has a positive function - find out what yours is.

3. What is the one thing/action I have not been willing to do that would cause me to achieve my weight loss goals'? Understand this: I did not say: "What have you not done that would cause you to achieve your weight loss goals." I asked you: " What are you not WILLING to do..."

Before you can really succeed in the weight game you must be willing to do absolutely anything necessary, including: give up chocolate; avoid alcohol, exercise four hours a day; study nutrition; bring your lunch to work; eat a bag of carrots at a wedding; meditate everyday and more... WAIT!!!!!!!!!!!!!!!!!!!!!! Please pick the book up off the floor and catch your breath. All I said was you have to be willing to do these things not that you would have to do them. Something magical happens when you commit to being willing to do whatever it takes to achieve your goals. Your attitude changes. I have met many, many people who tell me over and over again how desperately they have tried to lose weight and on and on. Sometimes they have made large mistakes in their weight loss strategy, (i.e. exercise methods, foods, etc.) but always they are unwilling to do or not do something that would make all the difference. This same strategy of being willing to do whatever it takes to achieve your goals can make you a millionaire, a movie star, or simply a very healthy, fit person. You must search within yourself for the answer. It does not have to be monumental. You may not be willing to avoid certain foods. You may not want to deal with advances from the opposite sex (or your spouse). You may not want to be thought of as "shallow" and only interested in your body. You may not have been willing to look feminine or masculine, and act aggressively. You must decide what it is for you and choose to be willing to do it anyway if you want to succeed. Realize all you have to do is one or two actions that are different from what you are doing now to achieve permanent, natural weight control. Those actions simply need to become habitual. Your habits will determine your success or failure. Develop good habits and live by them everyday. Later on you will learn a self-hypnosis technique to condition your mind until habit takes over.

TO BE OR NOT TO BE - OBSESSED...

I have seen and heard the stories of women who have lost as much as 185 lbs. and more. Many record everything they put in their mouths; write down every calorie consumed and weigh themselves daily sometimes twice per day. I may have described someone you know well. Anyone, yourself included, who has done this type of behavior has high self-discipline. Think about that for a moment: The behaviors of keeping track, writing down, weighing in, and more require self-control and discipline. Beware: You can also slip into obsession. Obsession is when your thoughts are constantly on food, your weight, fat, calories, and the like. (Compulsion is feeling compelled to perform an action.)

Discipline leads to Freedom; Obsession leads to Slavery:

Compulsion is characterized by words like: I have to; I must; I've got to; It has to. Discipline might also come in the form of those words, but freedom is contained in these words: I can; I will; I want to; I do not want to; I prefer. There is no doubt that high achievement will require language like, " I must go out and run right now" or "I have to run 6 times this week to reach my weight goals." This type of discipline is part of every successful life and is generally not compulsive. The important part is that you have to do certain actions because you want to achieve certain results - that is discipline with freedom.

Compulsion is without choice. Choice is freedom. Choice can mean discipline. Choice without discipline leads to being out of con-

trol. Imagine giving a four-year old complete choice without any discipline! Prolonged discipline without choice is obsession. Consider for your ultimate goal Discipline -with Choice.

This is the secret to having your cake and eating it too. You can have the desserts, and soda and alcohol. You must also realized the price to pay for being healthy, happy, fit, lean, energetic, strong, respected, admired, and even more attractive. It probably means avoiding those substances 29 days out of 30 (and loving it!) instead of 1 out of 2.

After you have disciplined yourself for sometime you may feel deprived. This is the "losing" way to think about it. You did not deprive yourself! You rewarded your body by giving it maximum nourishment and digestive rest! It will, it must, thank you for that with all the benefits of health and fitness. After substantial discipline take pride in your efforts. Self-discipline is something to be proud of. Feel it! Others will respect you for it. Even when you eat food that is fattening or not good for you - do it with self-control - do it with the mindset of.- " I am choosing to eat this!" Even if you feel compelled. Then maybe choose to exercise, or buy healthy food or walk a mile, you'll be amazed at how in control you feel. It is all about self-control - feeling in charge of you! Studies in stress management confirm that lack of control, that is, feeling out of control makes you feel stressed out. If stress is a major factor in your life you must take control of the situations that cause you stress. If you are reading this book, your weight is probably stressful to you. To take charge and reduce the stress your aim is to feel in control of your weight, health, body and energy. Every action you take that makes you feel more confident, more fit, more energized and more capable, makes you feel more in control and lowers stress levels. If you go out and run one mile, if that's challenging to you, you will feel better about yourself. You will feel more in control and the stress about your weight will decrease. If you do that every day, your fitness will increase, your weight will decrease along with your stress levels.

Consider your weight control experience as a journey, a test, a self-assessment that is giving you FEEDBACK; feedback that will make you better, stronger and more self-aware. Knowing yourself is important. However, I know many people who say, "Oh, I know I would never be able to give up coffee, I know myself." You were not born into this world drinking coffee or smoking or eating cookies, therefore, you learned to do it. Anything you learned to do, you can relearn and change or modify, and it can happen quickly. Think back to a time when you amazed yourself at what you were able to do after you did it. I am sure you have had a few, if not many, of those experiences. Remember them and use them as a source of inspiration.

FOODS and FEELINGS

I can remember sitting in many of the apartments I have lived in feeling like I had no one in the world I could relate to except Breyer's® ice cream and Chips O'Hoy® cookies! Somehow buying this junk food made me feel like I was doing something special for myself. I thought I would feel better - maybe I did for a short while, but not for long. You may be upset to hear that I never gained more than a pound or two from my junk food habit and you would never have noticed the gain. However, the issue was not the food but the feelings. I felt psychologically uncomfortable at certain times and took control. On most occasions I took control by exercising or eating very well. The problem arose when I felt deprived or I felt as if nothing special was happening to me so I made it a point to eat "special junk food." Fortunately for me these feelings were short-lived and I did spend more time being highly active versus eating junk. Many athletes do the same thing. It's detrimental and it does not solve the underlying feelings.

Your task is to identify the feelings that lead you to certain foods. Sadness, fear, anger, joy, happiness, anxiety, worry, frustration, disappointment, guilt, hurt, boredom overwhelm, loneliness, love, confidence, cheerfulness and any others. Do you eat more food or unhealthy food under the influence of any of these emotions? I am sure you do. Make a list of the emotions that trigger you toward unhealthy eating patterns.

There are two ways to deal with this type of "emotional eating:" (1) You can do psychological work and resolve the cause of the feeling and develop new emotional and behavioral patterns in order to feel and behave differently. Or (2), you can simply develop new behaviors when you feel these feelings. Everyone feels loneliness, but not everyone eats the whole house. Some people jog, or walk or call their friends and family or read or make it a point to go to social functions or public places and meet people. The same can be said of anger or any other emotion, every person deals with the emotion in either a long term supportive way or a long term detrimental way (i.e. resolving vs. overeating).

My suggestion is for you to use the number two (2) method for now. If you would like to use the number one (1) method, seek out a therapist trained in hypnosis or Neuro - Linguistic Programming (NLP) to help change your associations and patterns of behavior. Or you could study NLP or self-hypnosis and resolve issues within yourself.

Visualize yourself behaving the way you want to behave in tough situations with food. Imagine your body the way you want it to look. Do this when you awake in the morning and/or before you go to sleep at night. This is the time when your subconscious is more accessible and your conscious mind less critical. Visualization works. All great athletes use visualization, (consciously or subconsciously) on many different levels. The reason visualization works is very simple. Conscious and subconscious images (thoughts) in the mind influence the body internally and externally. The majority of that thought is subconscious - that is, below your conscious awareness of the thought. If your thoughts are driving your behaviors and those behaviors are producing your results, then you can control your results by controlling your thoughts. You control your thoughts best by taking charge of the pictures in your mind. That happens by imagination. The simplest way to use this power is: *Imagine going through your upcoming day. See your day in your mind the way you want it to be. When you do this you will increase the likelihood of it happening because you will be pre-programming your mind to act the way you want it to. Remember to enjoy this process. It is a process, never a static end result.*

There are many things to do to become lean and there are, of course, some not to do. Let's find out how to...

Chapter 6

Eat, Drink & Be Merry Strategy

"Let not your mind run on what you lack as much as on what you already have. Of the things you have select the best; and then reflect how eagerly they would have been sought if you did not have them."

— Marcus Aurelius Antoninus

Here it is. The part of this book you knew was coming. Food: I have never seen a more heated subject since the O.J. verdict! I meet with people of all types; executives, lean people, obese people, athletes and new mothers. The interesting thing is that virtually everyone tells me that they know what they should be eating. It never ceases to amaze me that everyone knows what to eat. However, after we have a few consultations it becomes clear that they could be eating much differently than they previously thought. I never stop learning about new foods, combinations and the new poisons the food companies try to feed us and I hope that you continue to educate yourself, too.

By choosing to avoid or drastically cut down on the following foods/substances you will lose weight and become much healthier. I HOPE THAT YOU USE THIS INFORMATION TO MAKE YOUR CHILDREN HEALTHY AND STRONG FOR THE FUTURE. Here we go:

Let me tell you what makes the **Living Lean!** program different from every other program out there: You should never be physiologically hungry when following the **Living Lean!** life-style of eating and drinking.

When I would meet with clients and explain to them the dietary program I had designed for them many would be very concerned that I was going to restrict their calories. Then I would tell them that I was not interested in calories and they shouldn't be either. What was important was food value. I would tell them they could typically eat as much as they wanted and that they should never feel hungry. Within a day or two I would hear, "John I am hungry - eating only 1 piece of fruit only lasts me for about an hour and then I get hungry again." At this point I gently tell them to eat much more. I remind them that they can eat as much as they want of fruit and juices in the morning (or anytime really). They often look confused at this point. I repeat what I have told them multiple times until it seems to have sunk in.

I say the same thing to you: never be hungry on this program - you don't need to be. In fact, I'll go one step further. You can eat all the junk food, all your favorite foods and all the foods I am going to tell you not to eat IF you will first eat and drink all the food and beverages I suggest you consume.

What you are being taught here are the principles of health and leanness. If I simply give you a list of behaviors you won't change your mind. Your mind is what is keeping you overweight or out of shape, because your actions are generated in your mind before they manifest in the physical world. By understanding the strategies in this program and integrating them into your life you will make them work for you. **Living Lean!** is like dancing. Once you know how to dance well you can just listen and feel the music and go with it. Once you understand the strategies in this program you will eat healthfully, exercise often, and avoid unhealthy foods almost automatically.

What follows are foods to eat very little of or totally avoid. It will do wonders for your health, your weight and your fitness levels.

1. **Meat:** Let me explain what I mean when I say meat. I mean anything with a face. That's right, all animals and fish: red meat, turkey, chicken, tuna and the like. You might be thinking, "You're crazy, I can't give up all of that - what else is there to eat, granola?!" Actually, granola is not that great of a food either, but seriously, let me explain. First of all, consider *reducing your intake* of these foods. Many people will eat three meals per day of these foods - it is mind boggling to me. Having bacon in the morning tuna or some fish for lunch and then steak or a hamburger for dinner. Now, you may not eat that, but be honest. Are you having hot dogs, hamburgers, fish, chicken, turkey, lamb, ham, cold cuts - on a daily or even two to three times per day basis? My guess is you are.

A friend of mine works in a hospital. Recently she attended a special presentation given by one of the medical doctors about the colon, fiber, and surgery. She couldn't believe the amount of fiber the doctors were telling everyone to consume. When I asked her what they said she could only say, "a lot!" At this presentation she and other personnel in the hospital were shown slides of the inside of patients colons. It was startling. I have personally seen photos of what has come out of peoples colons after detoxification therapies - and that is shocking. The amount of fecal matter that is packed in one's colon is incredible. Fecal matter from cooked foods, pasta, cheese, milk, meat, swallowed gum, and finger nails chewed and swallowed creates a very toxic substance inside the body. This substance can be as thick and hard as tire rubber. One case I read about described the unbelievable fact that 40 lbs. of fecal matter came out of one man's colon! It is not uncommon to have several pounds of fecal matter within the colon - stuck. Your colon is your most important organ for health and weight management. Your colon is the sewage system of your body; clean it out regularly if you want to be disease-free. Let it accumulate waste and you will certainly pay the price. Remember: "Death begins in the colon."

My friend was urged by the physicians presenting at the meeting to consume great quantities of fiber or else expect at some point, like many hospital patients, to have surgery to remove the waste and part of the colon (colostomy). The point of this is to recognize that meat is not fiber. Meat will usually take days, sometimes up to three days or more, to digest. It is likely that some of this meat will remain in the colon for extended periods of time - a perfect breeding ground for bacteria, even worms and parasites. This waste is just lying there, weighing you down. Consume more fiber daily and reduce your consumption of meat to one time per week or less.

Meat Is a Piece of Dead Corpse
(Harsh, but true)

If you would not kill the animal that you typically eat yourself, then, you should reconsider eating it at all, as a morality issue. From simply a health, fitness, and weight loss issue, meat is not really a healthy food. When an animal dies, putrefactive germs, germs from the animal's colon (do you remember what's in the colon?) saturate all the cells of the meat. It is putrefactive germs that tenderize the meat. Do you understand what you are eating?? There's more. In recent years, newspapers and big-time magazines (March 28, 1994 cover of Newsweek) have printed articles about antibiotics in our milk. How do antibiotics get into our milk? Farmers give the antibiotics to their animals.

Since 1950, antibiotics have been widely used to stimulate

the growth of young chickens, cattle, and pigs. It was found that low level antibiotics added to animal feed improved weight gain by 10 to 11 percent. The drugs are also used to increase egg production. Antibiotics are administered at higher levels in feed or drinking water or by injection in the treatment of various livestock diseases. Almost 50% of the antibiotics used in the United States are used for animals. The average person gets antibiotics in their food daily - up to 80 different drug traces have been found in the milk you get off the shelf. No wonder the effectiveness of prescribed drugs are declining on humans. The average person has built up a tolerance and new antibacterial "super " bacteria have built up a tolerance as well. This makes antibiotics almost useless on humans today. What you need to realize is this: before the drugs got into the milk it was in the animal and is still in all the tissues of the animal after it is killed. Ruth Winter, M.S. states in her book, Poisons in Your Food, that the antibiotics approved by the FDA for animal growth promotion include: bacitracin, bamemycins, chlortetracycline, erythromycin, lincomycin, monesin, oleandomycin, oxytetracycline, tylosin, virginiamycin and more. Milk is allowed to contain a certain concentration of 80 different antibiotics - all used on dairy cows to prevent udder infections. With every glassful people swallow a minute amount of several antibiotics. Farm animals receive 30 times more antibiotics than most people do.

Penicillin is being added to the feed and drinking water of salmon, catfish, lobsters, chicken, swine, and turkeys. What about hot dogs - glad you asked. Hot dogs are made from the most undesirable parts of the animal. They are colored in order to make them look pink or else the hot dog would be brown like the feces it's original organ helped eliminate. I suggest you avoid hot dogs. Do yourself and your children a favor - limit meat to once or twice per week or per month. Personally, I would never eat a hot dog, I'd rather eat ... let's talk about chicken.

The U.S. Department of Agriculture reports that about 37% of chicken carcasses carry salmonella. Four percent of all beef and 12% of all pork is also contaminated but chickens are coprophagous (they eat each others droppings) so salmonella is a common inhabitant in their intestinal tract. This information comes from Anthony

Robbins' <u>Living</u> <u>Health</u> program, which is a recommended program.

You may be thinking, "where will I get my protein?" Well, where do the elephant, cow, and rhinoceros get theirs? Vegetation. Fruits, vegetables and grains have substantial amounts of protein. Beans and soy are also good sources. Use spirulina, it's 60% protein and a near perfect food, unlike milk. You rarely have to concern yourself with whether you are getting enough protein or calcium. Dr. N.W. Walker, among others, has concluded that all essential amino acids are available in fruits and vegetables (see <u>The Vegetarian Guide</u> <u>to Diet and Salad).</u> These foods do not have to be combined in a special order as once thought. The average American gets twice the amount of protein he or she needs on a daily basis, yet they receive far below the nutritional requirements they need. The fear of too little protein is very psychological. It is one that has been imbedded into our minds since childhood. Many world champion body builders from ages 20 - 60 are vegetarians and are bigger and stronger than even the most enthusiastic weight trainer could hope for.

Besides, when do you think you need the most protein in your lifetime? That's right: when you are a newborn baby. Mother's milk provides the perfect amount - 1.2 - 1.6% protein. This amount of protein is similar to the amount found in fruit. Try cutting down on your protein and see for yourself. You will feel lighter because meat takes days even weeks to digest and you will have more energy because you aren't spending it on intense digestion. If you are concerned about your vitamin/mineral or protein intake consider taking supplements as suggested earlier for optimal health. Some people get uncomfortable when I recommend supplements to people without a doctor's prescription. Whenever you read a label that a food is fortified with certain vitamins it means the manufacturer has sprinkled vitamin powder into the vat containing the product. That is supplementation - no one seems concerned about that. Most people consider that a positive attribute in a food. The problem is not the supplementation of the food, it is the food itself. It is a dead food with a few vitamins sprinkled in to make it seem like you and I are really going to be healthy by eating it - good luck.

2. Dairy Products: Milk, skim milk, cheese, yogurt, are all dairy

products and are:

A. Difficult if not impossible to digest: Lactose intolerance, the inability to digest lactose because of a lack of the enzyme lactase, sets in at about 4 years of age. A reported 80% of people worldwide including most Africans, Greeks, and Asians (Nutrition concepts and controversies, by Hamilton, Whitney and Sizer) are affected. Some people will instead have an allergic reaction to the protein in milk. An allergic reaction can create an intense craving for the very food causing the allergy. I can personally say I had symptoms of a milk food allergy or intolerance years ago before I stopped drinking milk, and now I rarely eat any dairy products. As a result the symptoms which exacerbated asthmatic symptoms for me have stopped.

B. Milk neutralizes the hydrochloric acid (HCL) in the stomach. The body must work hard to produce more HCL in an attempt to digest the food. Eventually the glands producing HCL become exhausted and malabsorption of the nutrients occurs. Dairy tends to generate excessive mucus in the intestines, sinuses and lungs. This mucus will harden and form a coating on the inner lining which impedes nutrient absorption, the result - fatigue.

I suggest you avoid dairy. Also, the antibiotics we discussed before are in the milk, as well as the meat of the animal. Remember, those drugs were given not only to reduce disease, but primarily to promote faster, greater growth. The truth is, it will make you bigger too - not good for weight loss.

What about Calcium?

Many doctors I know tell their patients to take Tums® because it contains calcium and is cheaper than vitamins. I cannot tell you how repulsive this practice is to me. Drugs are not vitamins or minerals. Drugs are designed to do a masking of symptoms or kill organisms, not supply nutrients. Tums®, like any other drug can severely imbalance your body's acid - base production. Any doctor prescribing a drug to do the job of a vitamin or mineral is either bought out by a drug company or just ignorant of the body. Don't be just as ignorant, take a vitamin if you want to get a vitamin nutrient.

Or your other option is to eat the foods containing that vitamin in their whole form. Calcium (a mineral) can be gotten from green leafy vegetables. Calcium is found in broccoli, cabbage, carob, collards, dulse, figs, kale, oats, parsley, prunes, tofu, sesame seeds and other foods. Carrot juice has calcium in it therefore, drink it daily. I suggest a calcium-magnesium supplement. Calcium gluconate is recommended because it is usable, nontoxic up to 15,000 mg. and superior to bone meal, calcium chloride and calcium lactate.

Exercise and Your Bones

Probably most important, for the prevention of osteoporosis, is exercise. Exercise is much more important than taking calcium supplements. Yes, it is true that you need calcium throughout your whole life to have strong bones, but exercise will make bones stronger too. When you stop moving the body against resistance (i.e. when you are bedridden) the bones lose calcium fast. You will lose more calcium by not exercising against resistance (i.e. weight training, calisthenics, running, powerwalking, or intense bike riding are resistance exercises but swimming is usually not). Astronauts left in space for long periods of time will lose calcium because of the weightlessness (lack of resistance) in space. Their return to space is often a concern. Their skeletons may be too weak to support their weight from loss of calcium in the bones.

Start moving your body against resistance in order to maximize your bone density and protect yourself from osteoporosis. See our exercises in the back of the book.

3. Alcohol and Your Brain: For the people I have worked with cutting down on alcohol offered measurable weight loss. Avoid alcohol and you will lose weight in a timely fashion. If you have 2 drinks per day (about 300 calories) or so and then abstain, you will typically lose .5 - 1 lbs. per week. If you also consume snacks with the alcohol and avoid them, you'll lose more.

Alcohol has seven calories per gram. Fat has nine and carbohydrate and protein have approximately four calories per gram each. Forget everything you may have been told about alcohol having protein, supplying nutrients or energy. Recognize alcohol as the product of decay that it is. Here is what happens when alcohol is ingested.

Once in the stomach and small intestine, alcohol is absorbed directly into the bloodstream. Part of every sip of alcohol you take is absorbed right through your tongue and gums before you even have time to swallow it! Dr. Melvin H. Knisely and associates of the medical college of South Carolina warns, "every time a person takes one drink of alcohol - even a social one - he permanently damages his brain, killing off tens of thousands of brain cells." (see Living Health, by A. Robbins).

Alcohol, Knisely says, starts the blood cells clumping together causing the blood to become a thick sludge, slowing down the flow of oxygen to the brain. That is what causes that "high" feeling, a lack of oxygen in the brain. Knisely says, "whenever a social drinker has had enough to feel happy, he has begun to kill off his brain cells. A heavy drinking bout could damage as many as 100, 000 brain cells." As far as scientists know, the damage is permanent; however, recent studies suggest that brain cells can regenerate - a concept dismissed as impossible for decades. Alcohol is not a stimulant but a narcotic. It lessens endurance and one's resistance to disease. As far as preventing heart disease - exercise instead.

One other thing about alcohol. Extreme alcoholic intoxication can cause acute organic brain disorder at any age. Sometimes the organic disorder is not directly caused by alcohol, but by dietary deficiencies. Fredrick Hatfield, Ph.D. states in Ultimate Sports Nutrition, that alcohol blocks absorption of vitamins and washes them out of the body. Alcohol-related protein deficiency can lead to cirrhosis of the liver, a potentially fatal disease. Specifically, if vitamin B is deficient long enough it can lead to Korsakoff's syndrome, a chronic organic brain disorder. This syndrome is similar to Alzheimer's disease.

I have only touched on alcohol here. For weight loss, and health stop consuming it or cut it in half.

4. Coffee/Caffeine: Caffeine stimulates the adrenal glands putting the body into the "stress response". The stress response causes

hyper-alertness, tightened muscles, bladder discharge, blood sugar increase, nervousness and many more physiological changes. Chocolate, coffee and soft drinks often contain caffeine in addition to dairy, sugar and/or other chemicals.

In 1981 Dr. Brian MacMahon and colleagues at Harvard found that heavy coffee drinking was the only variable that separated 369 pancreatic cancer patients from 644 other patients. More than five cups per day brings a three times greater risk of cancer than no coffee at all. Decaffeinated is not a safe switch as far as cancer is concerned, because it is thought that caffeine is not the cause of cancer.

Avoiding coffee and caffeine may not directly influence your weight but it will improve your health. It can influence your weight for this reason: Coffee is acidic. Acid in the body attracts water to neutralize the acid. Excess water makes you heavier and bloated. Eliminate the acid and your body won't have the need to hold on to extra water.

Consider that the artificial stimulation from caffeine comes from creating a stress response in you, that is, stimulating the adrenal glands to release adrenaline. It can take the adrenal glands up to 24 hours to shut off once stimulated. Over time they can become exhausted and nonfunctional.

Like alcohol, avoid coffee and caffeine or at least cut your intake in half.

5. Junk Food, the Big Temptation: You must master your consumption of junk food. This can be difficult or even impossible until approached properly. The keys here are mindset, attitude and proper nutrition. The thought process that will ruin your success is the deprivation mindset.

The deprivation mindset is a major block to leanness. I was at a Spa in 1997 as a guest. I was there to reflect and to improve my health and fitness plan. The owner came in to greet a small group of us, most of whom wanted to lose weight. He looked at one woman who needed to lose about 100 lbs. and she introduced herself to him. He said, "you won't be eating while you're here. You need to lose weight." She looked a bit shocked and tried to stay cool and collected. I was feeling a bit uncomfortable for her. She did not eat for a few days, but pretty soon she and all the others who were-told "don't eat - just drink juices" were eating with the best of them. It was a kind of rebellion triggered by being deprived. The owner who has a Ph.D. in nutrition and psychology failed to understand this basic mindset that plagues so many overweight people.

I once worked with a woman whose goal was to be able to eat whatever she wanted, whenever she wanted, as much as she wanted. That's like the person who wants to become rich and do whatever he/she wants all the time. If you are super rich you can likely buy whatever you want at anytime. I know many wealthy people - they are basically conservative. I have known many fit people. The more fit they are the more careful they are with what goes into their body, usually. The reward of that discipline is that they can eat anything they want anytime, usually without any guilt over it. Just because they can does not mean they do. I know most people say that if they won millions they would buy expensive items and give some of the money to their friends, family, and associates. The truth is those who earn their money, rarely spend it carelessly.

That's part of the prosperity consciousness which is similar to the fitness mindset. The fitness state of mind never takes physical success for granted, but instead feels grateful for that success. The person who just worked out intensely and feels good is far less likely in most cases to go down and buy an ice cream cone. The reason is because they recognize that the ice cream with all the fat, sugar, diary products and anything else artificial, is going to slow down the fitness process they just spent one or two hours to develop. Does that make sense to you? If not you need to exercise more often. When a person works hard for their money and they relate to the fact that eight hours of hard work gives them $100 to put in their pocket, they are less likely to go out and spend $75 at the race track. Those who do, probably have a serious problem and they need to get help.

How do you acquire this fitness mindset? It may be a slow transition for you or it may happen quickly, either way, you can develop this mindset by:

1. Deciding who you want to be; how you want to look; how you want to feel everyday and what that will mean about you and to you.

75

For example, "I want to be an inspiration to young children; or my employees; to look strong; to feel energetic; it means I am 'strong' or 'loving' and that I care about myself."

2. Start. Take consistent action each day. Even if you're out of town on business take a few minutes to do some stretches at least. This will keep your mind focused on your fitness goals.

Personally, the way I eat today is very different from how I ate ten years ago. Ten years ago I was eating: 2 - 3 bowls of cereal with whole milk (or 2% milk) in the morning, a meat or tuna sandwich or pizza with milk for lunch, 2 - 4 peanut-butter sandwiches around mid to late afternoon, and maybe pasta or more peanut butter sandwiches for dinner (with milk or juice). I did eat fruit and vegetables. Usually it was a token vegetable on the side of the plate or convenient fruit near by. I was strongly addicted to dairy products. My addiction to dairy was so strong and irrational that even when experiencing an asthma attack, and knowing milk would make it worse, I had to have it anyway. Of course, the milk made more mucus and increased my coughing.

The truth is that soda, candy, gum, pizza, cookies, cake, ice cream and anything with lots of sugar is going to ruin your health, your teeth and your chances at weight loss. Your body is likely to turn the simple carbohydrate (sugar) into fat and store it on your body in adipose tissue (fat cells).

I know I am giving you all of this information at once. Cold turkey is usually the most effective way to change behaviors. You may need to reduce your coffee intake by half each week for a month. Or you may need to do the same thing with dairy. That is certainly all right to do. Make sure you don't kid yourself by saying, " well, I only use a little milk in my coffee" or "I eat the 'no fat' cookies." Go all the way. I started to cut down butter by putting less and less on bread. Finally, I got to the point where I did not need or even want any butter. You can too. Kidding yourself about how "little" sugar, fat, dairy, coffee, etc. you eat is the surest way to end up eating all the foods the food industry makes hundreds of billions of dollars each year selling you. Don't be manipulated by the food industry.

Decide to take charge of your health and what you put into your mouth. You might want to go to a local health food store in your area and buy the healthier food it has. If you don't have one - consider starting your own health food business. With the internet it is more possible to do than ever.

Question: " I've done this sort of thing before and it tends to get expensive doesn't it?

Answer: I have heard that before. If you continue buying junk food and health food, then yes it will. If, however, you replace the foods you were eating with fruits, vegetables, grains like couscous, and quinoa (keen -wa), amaranth (these two are high in protein and are wheat - gluten free) you will pay the same or less for your food. Only if you eat junk food and healthy foods together will it get costly. Go to the cupboard and calculate the cost of all the meats, fish, dairy, junk food and coffee you buy. If you are average at all it's practically your entire refrigerator. If you buy food for others in your house as well, give them this book and tell them the reasons you are buying different foods. Ask them to either buy their own food or try what you are buying. It's your body and your life - why compromise?

Question: I really don't eat much junk food just 1 or 2 cookies a day - that's not bad is it?

Answer: This is a mindset problem. You need to master those cookies by mastering your false need to have them everyday. You might be better off if you saved up the cookies all week and ate 7 or 14 of them at once. Other than that, junk food creates vitamin deficiencies and metabolic, circulatory and cardiac abnormalities. Dr. Michael Colgan and associates of Rockefeller University, have measured these functions on subjects and found that it takes 72 hours to return to normal. If you are eating them daily you are creating a chronic state of abnormal function.

A study Colgan conducted had both athletes and overweight subjects restrict processed fat in their foods for three days. They were then allowed a one day binge. Then they avoided the processed foods for another three days. The binge-restrict cycle was seven days long. All ate far more calories on the binge day than they had cut out of their diets during the restricted period. However, they lost weight consistently. Even the athletes lost three to five pounds during the four-week study and they were lean to begin with. Why? The body has a limited capacity to digest sugars and starches at any one time. Therefore, not all the calories will be absorbed, but excreted. Eating a little junk at a time will allow the body to digest, absorb and store nearly all the calories. Caution: if your body is highly trained to store fat (if you can pinch more than four inches on your waist it's trained to store fat!) then you will store much more of the calories than the lean metabolism person.

EAT a LOT of JUNK FOOD

If you are going to eat non-healthy food then allow yourself one day per week to do it. This is a psychological tactic too. You'll have something to look forward to and the guilt factor will be eliminated or greatly reduced. Challenge yourself to wait until Saturday or whatever day you choose to have your binge on. I use the word binge to mean simply eating somewhat more than you would normally eat at one time.

I had been using this strategy for many years before I knew of a physiological basis for it. I have also found that people with the toughest weight conditions eat a little junk everyday. My suggestion to you is cut it out completely or limit yourself to one "fun day" where you eat what you want.

How about a type of food to eat much more of? Here it is:

FIBER: Fiber consists of many compounds, mostly carbohydrates. These compounds are indigestible in the intestine and give bulk to the intestinal contents. Lack of fiber leads to disease: Some of the diseases that can occur from too little fiber include: cancer, diverticulosis, atherosclerosis, and others. Ten years ago the scientific nutrition books were saying that although eating more fiber was a good idea, and that countries who ate high fiber diets do not contract the diseases mentioned above and those that eat less fiber (Western countries) do contract the diseases, it still did not prove that low fiber leads to disease. Ten years later no one argues with eating a large amount of fiber for health. Here's the point: Your doctor will tell you to exercise, but he won't tell you how or about cardiovascular or weight training exercise - he's too busy and it's not his expertise. He will tell you to eat properly, but not how. He won't tell you about raw food, or to avoid meat as much as possible. What you are reading in this book is years ahead of what you will hear on prime time news or in most magazines. You don't have to wait to learn cutting-edge strategies for health and fitness. Take advantage of it by using it today.

Fiber promotes weight loss by creating a feeling of fullness. You eat less food and fewer calories. You also move fecal matter, which has weight, out of your body. Fiber relieves constipation by attracting water into the digestive tract, softening stools and relieving the intestinal pressure that could lead to hemorrhoids. Fiber keeps the intestinal contents moving regularly thus, preventing bacterial infection of the appendix (appendicitis). Fiber stimulates the muscles of the digestive tract so that they retain their health and tone preventing diverticulosis in which the intestinal walls become weak and bulge out in places.

Fiber binds fatty compounds (sterols) and carries them out of the body in the feces so that blood cholesterol concentration is lowered and most likely the risk of heart and artery disease is too. How much fiber do you need per day? I'll give you a conservative number: 15 - 30 grams of dietary fiber. 25 grams of fiber would be:

*1 apple
*2 plums and
*1 peach

That is the minimum each day. Other sources include: Wheat bran, oat bran, raw vegetables, raw fruits, psyllium husk. Again, it is perception. You are not on a diet, you are choosing a life-style to live your life by. If you have kids, teach them to live this way, they will be healthier for it. You probably don't give much thought to the next principle, but it is very important for your health. It is very simply...

Chapter 7

The Water & Weight Loss Strategy

"Do whatever you can do and as much as you can do at the time. Any amount of practice is better than no practice at all"

— *Hidy Ochiai*

Karate Master

It has been reported that underground water, your *drinking water*, is the most dangerous pollution problem in America. The Environmental Protection Agency (EPA) has reported 55,000 chemical dump holes across the nation which can leak their contents into the groundwater. The EPA has established a firm link between chlorinated tap water and created carcinogenic compounds called trihalomethanes. Trihalomethanes are associated with cancer of the kidney, urinary tract, bladder, lymph nodes and brain. Solution: Do not drink tap water, but before you buy just any bottled water - be warned. Labels reading: "Spring Pure" or "Natural Spring Fresh" are usually just filtered tap water. It is no better than your tap water. Buy (steam) distilled water, it's pure. You do not want anything in your water - not chlorine, not fluoride, not minerals - NOTHING!

Your life began in water and your body and earth are mostly water. Water is a big part of our world. Water is part of the chemical structure making up cells, tissues and organs of the body. Considered the universal solvent, water moves nutrients and waste products through the body. Water acts as a lubricant around joints and protects sensitive tissue around the spinal cord from shock. Water also lubricates the digestive tract and all tissues moistened with mucus.

Many people are often dehydrated. You can tell if you are taking in enough water by the color of your urine. Bright or dark yellow urine is too concentrated; you need more water. Pale yellow, almost colorless urine is dilute enough, your water intake is ample. Some supplements will turn your urine a bright color - it's harmless. Gary Null, Ph.D. in his book *Gary Null's Ultimate Anti-Aging Program*, recommends drinking one gallon of purified water per day. Common sense says that youthful plants and humans are filled with water. Old and dying plants and humans are dehydrated and dry. Make drinking one gallon of water per day a goal, and replace the coffee and alcohol you consume with pure, energy promoting water. If you are consuming fresh vegetable and fruit juice, they have pure water within them. Each glass counts towards your overall water intake for the day.

Alcohol and coffee tend to dehydrate a person. Water will transport toxins out of your body as urine, fecal matter and perspiration. The message is clear: Drink Enough Water! You will get water through fresh fruits and vegetables, as well as by drinking distilled water. Drink before you become thirsty; thirst indicates you are already dehydrated. Again, you can double check this by the color of your urine.

To lose excess water weight you will need to drink more water. Your body will hoard whatever it thinks it is being deprived of. Therefore, going into a sauna to sweat off weight will work until you drink fluids with water - then the body draws the water in and holds on to it. Consider taking the supplements listed earlier to help rid the body of excess water.

BONUS INFORMATION: Some of the people I have worked with who use oral contraceptives or estrogen replacement drugs have had difficulty losing weight after the first five or ten pounds. All drugs have side effects - all of them. Drugs are poisons to the human body. Sometimes they are necessary poisons. Otherwise, consider alternative methods for contraception and estrogen replacement. I realize some readers will resist the blanket statements I make about drugs. Realize that you can, most likely, achieve the same or similar results by taking natural herbal remedies, instead of drugs. I strongly suggest you look into it. The herbal remedies rarely have the side effects and are safer overall with exceptions - like everything in life. For example, ephedra must be taken with great care.

Your goal in this program is to lose fat, get rid of toxic fecal matter weighing you down and blocking the absorption of nutrients, and retrain your biochemistry (enzymes, muscle cells and blood) to burn fat efficiently. One important change to make in order to achieve your goals and do it in a fun way is to use your mind and …

Chapter 8

Master Stress & Relax Your Way To Weight Loss Strategy

"Be kind, for everyone you meet is fighting a hard battle."
— Plato

Stress is still a buzz word. The reason, I believe, is simply because you and I have more complex tasks to do and evaluate everyday. The inability to reduce, manage and transform stress creates the stress response.

The stress response identified by Dr. Hans Selye (Cell - Yeah) is the fight or flight mechanism in the mind, body and nervous system. Being threatened physically causes us to go into the stress response. We either fight or flee. In our modem society we don't usually find ourselves in true life threatening situations very often. We do find ourselves in ego threatening situations once, twice, sometimes 10x a day. This creates enormous tension in the body, mind, and nervous system.

What I want to do here is give you fundamental knowledge about stress and how it affects your weight, and how to control it. I conduct stress management seminars for the general public and corporations. I have experienced many types of stress myself including, physical, mental, emotional, chemical and environmental stress. 75% - 90% of all doctors visits are for stress related conditions. According to The Institute of HeartMath, 72% of American workers experience frequent, stress-related physical or mental conditions that greatly increase health care costs. Forty percent of employee turnover is due to stress. One million employees per day are absent from work due to stress-related disorders. A 20-year study conducted by the University of London School of Medicine has determined that un-managed mental and emotional reactions to stress present a more dangerous risk factor for cancer and heart disease than cigarette smoking or eating high cholesterol foods. Read that last study again and grasp the importance of it.

What this means to you is that negative stress (dis-stress) about your weight, your money, your health, your job or anything else, can cause you very serious health problems and prematurely age your body and mind, as well. Notice how much most presidents seem to age after only four years in the White House. Who do you know who has gone through very stressful experiences and has become older more quickly.? The chemicals that flood into the body during the *fight or flight response* cause damage to the body when this response happens too often. While the stress response is the same for everyone the actual behaviors you do when stressed vary from person to person.

Everyone has behaviors they do when under stress. Whether overweight or not, many people use food, drugs, and alcohol to distract themselves from anxiety, worry and stress. Besides the havoc stress plays on your adrenal glands and other bodily systems, many people find that stress causes them to feel time pressure and the need to eat. If you feel time pressure you will eliminate the first thing that does not seem urgent to you. Exercise is seldom urgent - like a phone ringing - but is it important? Of course it is. Your **Living Lean!** strategy then, must be to dedicate four to seven (4-7) days (forget two or three) to exercise even just 20 minutes each time, preferably more, twice per day. For example, fast walking to and from work or once at lunch and once before or after work. If it seems impossible you may have to seriously review your priorities in life. Do you want to make exercise a lifelong "habitual ritual" or not? Exercise will enhance the quality of your life. You'll feel better, and have more energy.

Next is food. The way to handle this stress distracter technique is with this *Master Stress Strategy:* Choose to give in to your desires once per week or month (yes we mentioned this before as a way to lose weight). The rest of the time have fruit, organic vegetables (organic is grown with fewer pesticides), plain rice cakes, buy organic carrots, or grapes (they aren't fattening) to munch on to keep your blood glucose level even. Foods that are full of preservatives, chocolate, sugar, or other sweeteners will often cause distress in your system. For example, coffee will stimulate your adrenal glands putting you into the stress response immediately. The greatest source of stress however, is our continual thoughts.

MENTAL STRESS CONTROL

I had never been on a subway train until I moved to New York City. I learned quickly that once I was inside the train I was at the mercy of the conductor. I could not open the doors once closed; I could not slow or speed up the train - nothing. One time on the train going into New York I noticed I was late for a meeting. Then suddenly the train just stopped. I had no idea why we stopped or how long we would be stopped. I felt trapped like a caged animal. This was the start of my stress control lesson. I learned that I had one question I had to ask myself. "Is this event controllable or uncontrollable?" The answer was uncontrollable. Since it was uncontrollable, I only had one choice: acceptance. If the situation had been controllable then I would have two choices: Take action and create the result that I wanted (I suppose I could have tried to break through the glass door and climb out onto the platform, as if I were Rambo, but I didn't) or consider the situation uncontrollable and accept it.

Those are your choices as well. Pick the situations that generate stress for you and decide if they are controllable or uncontrollable and take the appropriate action. One anxiety producing stressor for the majority of people is "uncertainty".

What if someone you know called you up and said, "hey, I've got bad news, but I'll call you tomorrow and tell you." That would probably drive you crazy with anxiety. How do you feel after you take an important test? You probably want to know how you did immediately and the suspense is maddening. We all tend to feel stressed when we are in uncertain situations. The answer to solving *uncertainty is* to resolve how you will feel and respond in any situation if it were to happen. Role play how you will respond and feel if you fail the test. How will you feel and how will you bounce back if you don't make the sale? This strategy will give you greater self-confidence and most importantly, *peace of mind.*

My strategy for peace of mind is to take time each day at the end or in the beginning, to be thankful for the chance to be alive for another day; to be grateful for the opportunity to enjoy myself, to contribute to other people and have relationships with the other people in my life. The fact that I'm *alive, free* and *healthy* really is soothing to me. If I didn't have my health or freedom I'd soon discover the other things in life that I'm grateful for. What are you grateful for? Think about it once a day and you'll start to increase your peace of mind bit by bit until you realize that everything beyond health and freedom is "icing on the cake." Even if you lost a loved one, lost money, lost an opportunity, or lost your physical ability you can have peace of mind. How, you ask? By acknowledging the enjoyment or value with what you had at one time and then putting the past behind you and focusing on what you want and what you have now that's great. If life is stressing you out, think about how you want life to be better. If you are saying, "well, if I had more money..." or "if I had a lover..." or "if I could lose 30 lbs..." you are telling yourself you won't be happy until something else happens. Be happy now with what is good in your life and work to make the part that is dissatisfying better. If you really won't be happy "until" take action now to make it better.

Take an hour, maybe a few hours early in the morning or later at night and sit down in silence. Ask yourself what kind of life-style you want to have. I mean, describe how you want your day to go from the time you wake up to the time you go to sleep. Where do you want to be, what do you want to do, who do you want to be with? If you're happy you can't be stressed out. Focus on doing what you want now or as soon as you possibly can. Why? Because happiness is in the doing. Ask any good athlete. The best athletes enjoy practice, enjoy playing, they enjoy it all, because that's where the challenge is. To me winning the game of life is about having an enjoyable time, accomplishing what I set out to do, and leaving something for others that will enhance their lives somehow (maybe this book). Being lean is great. Enjoying becoming lean and staying lean is better. Eating healthfully is good. Enjoying the process of cleansing and strengthening the body and mind is a rush. Being rich is great. Making money and doing what you enjoy to make the money is a thrill. So there it is. The key to achieving the body you want. Check out your life-style. Do what you can to start living the kind of life you want now, before you win the lottery. I think most people are really not that far away from how they really want to spend their lives, they only need to understand what they want to spend the major parts of their time doing each day and commit themselves to doing it now.

Pick A Method That Works For You And Make Time For It: When I went to see Bill Moyers with Charlie Rose at a live seminar in New York City years ago, Moyers said, "I don't have time to meditate, I'm very busy, but I make time each day for 20 minutes." He is sold on stress reduction in the form of meditation. Find a method that works for you. Your exercise time plus five minutes for concentration, meditation, breathing or prayer could do it for you.

Control: This book is about taking charge of your weight and your life. When you understand that message at your core you will be able to accomplish your most important goals.

Essi Systems, a San Francisco-based stress-research consulting firm has demonstrated new information on the relationship between *personal power* and stress. They found diet, physical fitness, being a nonsmoker and weight control, have a negligible effect on a person's ability to cope with <u>work pressures or rapid change.</u> The only factor out of 21 stress-related factors that could predict who became sick and who stayed healthy in work situations with high amounts of pressure was *personal power. Personal power* was feeling in control of one's time, resources, important information, work load and the like.

The opposite of personal power is feeling victimized or out of control. While diet and exercise may reduce your stress levels a small amount in work situations, <u>the real power with diet and exercise is making you feel in control of yourself.</u> When you take charge of your health and fitness you can use this feeling of strength and control to take charge of other aspects of your life. What aspect of your life do you need to take charge of now?

Now we are going to discuss one of the most popular pseudo-stress reduction methods in America and perhaps around the world; pull up a chair let's...

Chapter 9

Watch The Television Strategy

"The healthy and the wealthy are wise enough to limit their television viewing. I suggest you do the same."
— John Farley

The average person in the United States watches (has the television on) about three - six hours per day (some sources say seven hours). I find that amazing. Years ago I had a friend of a friend stay with me for one month. He would come over after work at about 6pm and turn on the television. He would watch it through dinner and then all night. He would fall asleep around midnight with the television still on - every night. I would end up turning it off at 2 or 3 o'clock in the morning. If I didn't wake up and turn it off it would stay on until he got up in the morning. Either way, he would watch another 1 1/2 hours in the morning (he worked as an engineer at NBC). He literally wasted 6+ hours everyday on television. That's an enormous amount of time. A person could exercise, cook and eat dinner, relax, read a book, listen to musical, educational or motivational cassettes or go out and network for business, play with their kids, or basically have a life.

When it comes to weight loss, the television is not your friend. Consider what happens when you sit in front of the television. You are sitting doing nothing, barely moving a muscle. Your metabolism slows more and more the longer you sit. Watching something educational might be acceptable, but most people watch programs that will in no way help them to improve the quality of their lives. I will grant you that silly, funny or just "interesting" shows are good entertainment and can sometimes be a form of stress reduction. The problem comes in when most of your week is filled with useless programs.

That is not the worst part for those wanting to decrease the body fat. Every 15 minutes we are bombarded with commercials. These commercials are primarily selling food. Advertisers are using every sensory channel to persuade you to eat their food. They show you their food with bright colors, people looking and sounding excited at the thought of eating the manufacturer's food and, of course, they tell you how great they feel the moment they taste the food. Commercials are always louder than the regular program you are watching and designed to get you emotional about the product. Sitting and watching is a trigger for food consumption, as well. The more time you spend in front of the television the more food you will likely consume.

Studies show that watching television is very strongly linked to obesity. It is probably making you gain more weight than anything else in your home. Michael T. Murray, N.D., states in, <u>The Complete Book of Juicing,</u> information from *Pediatrics* magazine, that the number of hours spent watching television is the strongest predictor for becoming obese! In fact, the August 4, 1999 *New York Times* article stated that children under 2 years old should not watch television, older children should not have television sets in their bedrooms and pediatricians should have parents fill out a "media history," along with a medical history, on office visits, according to recommendations by the American Academy of Pediatrics. Television can cause mental, social and physical health problems for young people. *Common sense says, stop watching the stupid, mind-numbing, violent shows and put on educational and inspirational programs.*

I used to be addicted to television for most of my life. Television is truly addictive. When you stop watching it for a while you will likely go through withdrawal symptoms. Believe me, go without television for one week if you can and when you watch it again in one week you will be so turned off by the commercials you may "mute" them like I do. You do not have to avoid television completely, simply plan it like you do the rest of the activities in your day. Decide to do what is important in your life instead of getting caught up watching television. The less you watch the less you are likely to eat junk and the more weight you will lose. Also, the food you eat when you watch t.v. is rarely healthful, it is usually crunchy junk food. The truth is...

JUST BY TURNING OFF THE T.V. YOU WILL LOSE WEIGHT!

Television also dulls the mind. It makes you and your children passive recipients of mental junk food. Success comes through action not watching others live out fantasy lives while your life passes by. Not all television is bad, some is very good and like everything, moderation is the key.

This book is not a quick gimmick, or some watered down

piece of advice from Richard Simmons (although, I do like Richard Simmons). This program is a blueprint,. I know can transform your body, your attitude, and your life-style. Taking care of yourself, respecting and caring about yourself enough to optimize your potential is my goal for you. If not for yourself, apply the concepts in this book so that your children will get the best information on health. Don't let them be manipulated by the food industry and cultural propaganda.

Some people have told me they are compulsive and obsessive and this program just won't work for them. Others just tell me they don't have what it takes to accomplish all of what's in this book. They aren't disciplined enough, they are too old, too busy at work, they have children and a spouse who don't agree with this program, they hate exercise, they can't drink vegetable juices, they get nauseous if they take vitamins, they work in a television store, they have to eat meat because they own a slaughterhouse, they won't eat fruit because they refuse to "stay near a bathroom" just in case years of constipation comes out, and of course, they just don't have enough time anyway.

Others have told me this book has changed their lives. The combination of research, **Living Lean!** strategies, inspirational stories and common sense is what it took for them to get their life together and get in shape.

It all comes down to priorities. How important is your ability to move, to stay looking young, to be a good role model for your friends or family, to avoid disease, and really live your life to the absolute fullest? As Stephen Covey says, "don't prioritize your schedule, *schedule your priorities.*" This book is about your mind as much as, if not more than, your body. Take care of your mindset and your body will practically take care of itself. It's not important where you start, but *that you* start, - and where you're going! To guarantee you success on your quest for a lean, energized body all you have to do is recognize...

Chapter 10

The Start Of Success Strategy

"The quality of a person's life is in direct proportion to their commitment to excellence, regardless of their chosen field of endeavor."

— Vince Lombardi

Legendary Football Coach

I have seen it so many times with athletes and in business people. It is a factor in weight management and fitness. It is important for excellent grades and financial success. If you have it success is not guaranteed, but if you don't have it you will fall short of your potential. What is this important ingredient? It is *commitment*. <u>Commitment is the one factor that is the starting point to your achieving what you want.</u> I use to say that discipline was the fundamental key, but before discipline can happen, a commitment must be made. Commitment means "to pledge to a position on some issue." Most people today are uncommitted. Those who are committed are often committed to the wrong things. What would you say about someone who is committed to watching Monday night football, but can't find time to exercise? What about the person committed to their job despite the fact that their spouse is getting ready to leave them? What about the teenager who is committed to doing drugs and skipping school? Your commitments and the level of those commitments will determine what you accomplish and the quality of your life.

When members of the Swedish national badminton team were asked what was the main difference between them and others who did not make the national team, their response was commitment. They said, "they wanted it more", "being willing to train harder and longer."

Test your commitment to anything right now. How committed are you to achieving your fitness goals? (Decide what they are first if you haven't done so already). One (1) means you have no commitment to the goal - it is not important to you. Ten (10) means it is the most important thing in your life.

1   2   3   4   5   6   7   8   9   10

Top winning athletes, according to Sports Psychologist Terry Orlick, rank their commitment to their sports 9 or 10. If you find your commitment to your fitness goals less than a nine (9), that is all right. Your commitment, even if it is a four (4), will increase. The key to becoming more committed is to take action, and keep your mind on your goals and your reasons for desiring those goals.

Arnold Schwarzenegger has said that one of his keys to

success was to decide on his goal and then just do whatever actions were necessary to accomplish it. Said another way, decide that you want something, and that it is important to you. Then, decide that you will go after it until you accomplish it. What if time was not a factor? Often we say to ourselves, "I will commit to this goal for one month and then if I haven't achieved it I'll go after something else."

Imagine what it would be like if you decided you wanted something and that you would keep after it until you achieved it. What will stop you from making this level of commitment is your fear of failure. This fear will cause you to doubt yourself. You start to think, "what if three years goes by and I haven't gotten there?" By focusing on what you want and why you want it and what it will mean to you to achieve it, you will be committed to your success.

Now, suppose you make this commitment. You are Mr./Ms. committed. You workout, eat right - you do it all. Somehow you never get where you want to go. You sabotage yourself just as you get close to achieving what you say want. This happens to athletes, lawyers, business people, salespersons, and weight loss enthusiasts.

I experienced the fear of success for a long time and in many situations. When I was about fifteen I was training in karate with my teacher. I was called over during the class to demonstrate my techniques to him. Then I was told to go back and join the rest of the class. At the end of the class, to my surprise, I was promoted to blue belt (about halfway to black belt). At the end of the class I said to him that I didn't think I was ready for the promotion and thanked him anyway. He let me know in no uncertain terms that he was the master. "If I want you to be a white belt you're a white belt. If I want you to be a black belt you're a black belt. If I want you to be a blue belt, you're a blue belt!" "Yes sir!" I said. Even though the highest ranking teacher in our style, an eighth degree black belt, author, five (5) time national champion, world renown karate master from Japan had promoted me, somehow I felt like I wasn't good *enough*. That is fear of success using perfectionism as a cover. Trying to be perfect stops satisfaction in an accomplishment and is a way to avoid progressing. Fortunately, I overcame this mental limitation.

The fear of success causes you to doubt your skills, and stop yourself from accomplishing your goals. A fear of success can be caused by the belief that if you achieve this goal or accomplishment you will be worse off than if you didn't. You may think, "my friends will not believe I'm that good," or "if I lose weight I'll be expected to keep it off'", or "if I lose weight and then gain it back it will be even worse because I put in all that time and effort." These thoughts and others that tell you "being a success is worse than not being a success" means that fear of success is a factor for you. Some people fear success because they don't want to stand out in a crowd. To be seen as special or different would be negative. Too much attention, too much perceived pressure or something similar. Yes, it is true that if you had a great body you would stick out (but certain body parts would stick out less) but convince yourself that it would be positive not negative. Mediocrity means not sticking out; it means being average, just like most people. In a crowd of successful people, the mediocre stand out like a whale on the beach.

To succeed you will have to choose success, and success is not mediocrity it is excellence. Most people fail because they are not willing to tell themselves they want to win and that they deserve to win. With weight loss and fitness, the reason you deserve to have the body and the energy you want is simple: you are going to work for it. Just as you deserve to get paid for the work you do on your job, you deserve to reap the rewards from your efforts in the gym and in the kitchen.

Remember, to end fear of failure make a commitment to continue toward your goal until you get there. To do this decide that your goal is something you really want. To end fear of success decide that you deserve to have this success and that life will be better in every way and in no way worse. If you are having trouble with either of these change the way you think - it is all a product of your mind.

Commitment is not the only key to success in your life, but it is the beginning of success, without commitment you will not achieve what you are capable of, especially in health and fitness. If you are having difficulty relating to the concept of commitment this may help: remember the first time you ever jumped off the high dive at the pool? I remember my first time. I climbed up the ladder to the diving board which was about ten feet above the water. It looked like it was very far down to the water. I was very anxious. I kept standing at the edge of the board trying to decide if I would jump or not. Each time I thought I would, I chickened out. People down below waiting for their chance to dive in were yelling, "just jump!"

Finally, the lifeguard told me to jump in. I now felt the do or die pressure and I jumped! It was scary and even when I hit the water it wasn't over; I had to swim to the top and to the side of the pool. That type of commitment involves overcoming your initial fears. It would be like joining a health club and putting the money down. It is a start, but you do have to do more than that.

Long term commitment is similar to making it through high school. You know you are going to finish, one way or another. College is a better example. You have no idea what the courses, the teachers, the examinations or even the life-style will be like. In spite of that you decide where you want to go and you go! You deal with the challenges as they come up. You are committed to graduating with your degree. Do the same with your weight loss and fitness goals and you will accomplish them much faster and easier.

The key to making commitment work is to imagine the kind of person you will be having accomplished your goal. With high school or college you imagined yourself, at some level, as a graduate - you knew you would achieve it and *be* a graduate. Do the same with fitness. Imagine the result you want. Image it fully in your mind. See it, and feel it completely. Do this over and over again until you become convinced and mildly obsessed with achieving it. The feeling you will have is similar to when you knew you were going to get something you wanted, it was just a question of exactly when.

A key to accomplishing your ultimate weight and fitness goals is using the full focus of your mind to your advantage. With your mind directing your body you will achieve success. There is one ancient mind tool that has helped more people accomplish their goals than any other that I can think of, it is...

Chapter 11

The Power Of Hypnosis Strategy

"Rule your mind, or it will rule you."
— Horace

I had read books on mind power when I was a teenager. _Think and Grow Rich With Peace of Mind_ by Napoleon Hill, was the first. I had been reading about martial arts masters and how they did incredible feats supposedly through mind power. Finally, I started learning about hypnosis. I read, studied, trained, practiced, failed, succeeded, and repeated the process over and over. After ten years of using hypnosis to help people remove warts, stop smoking, control weight, walk on fire, eliminate phobias and much more, I make the following statement: When done properly, hypnosis is an invaluable tool for success and achievement.

Hypnosis allows the person being hypnotized to go beyond the conscious mind to the subconscious mind. Imagine an iceberg with 9% of the iceberg above water and 91% below the surface. So it is with the conscious mind and the subconscious mind. The subconscious mind is the 91% below the surface, the part that remembers how to walk and talk without even trying. The subconscious mind remembers how to drive a car and eat at the same time. It also makes a person eat when they don't consciously want to, or smoke when they consciously try to stop or sabotage their success even though they say they want to succeed.

By using the power of the subconscious mind habits can change, feelings can change, perceptions can change. That is real power. If you can change how you feel, how you consistently behave, and how you perceive yourself and your world, you can change any aspect of your life. Some people are able to change these parts of their lives (feelings, habits and perceptions) consciously. We are all able to do it with some aspects of our lives. If weight loss has been a repeated problem for you, then you need to change your subconscious mind in order to achieve what you want.

I have spent years working with the best hypnotists I could find. I worked with Mike Tyson's hypnotist John Halpin (when Tyson was a 16 year old up and coming boxer, Halpin hypnotized him before his fights), I studied with Richard Bandler of Neuro-Linguistic Programming fame, and other hypnotherapists who had been using the skills for 15 - 30 years. After working with people in various areas and on myself for years here is what you need to know about hypnosis to make it work for you…

1. Hypnosis can and will help you direct your subconscious mind toward a goal. This is very powerful and more effective than simply telling yourself consciously "I want to be thin." The reason hypnosis is more effective is because your subconscious mind will direct your habitual thoughts and actions.

2. If hypnosis has failed you it is likely because you have not resolved beliefs within you that are in conflict. For example, you want to lose weight but fear the new style of eating will create problems within your family or with your friends. Another example is, you want to look great, but fear you will attract members of the opposite sex and you won't be able to resist the temptation. The temptation that you fear acting on may jeopardize your current relationship. Hypnosis is definitely effective at resolving these issues; however, you will need a competent hypnotherapist to work with you and it will most likely take a minimum of five sessions.

3. Hypnosis can break bad habits and reinforce positive habits. Babies have a lot of difficulty getting the fork into their mouths. They have to concentrate very hard. Adults never miss! If you were to hypnotize yourself over and over you could start to poke the fork into your nose. The point is, habits are psychophysiological, but they can be broken and relearned in a short amount of time.

For our purposes here, it would make the most sense for you to direct your subconscious mind toward the image of the person you most want to be like. Your mind is already directing your habits and body toward an image. That image may not be something you consciously decided that you wanted. To change that image you need to consciously decide what image you want to see and then put that new image into your subconscious mind. Once in your subconscious mind, the subconscious will direct your thoughts, feelings and actions toward accomplishing that image in your reality.

One way to do this is to read and look at magazines with pictures of people with bodies you admire and would be very happy to look like. You need to find yourself saying, "yeah, that's the type of body I want to have!" It needs to be an image that inspires you.

Inspiration is the best word to capture the feeling you want to have. When something inspires it motivates and excites. Once you have this picture of the body you really want to have, then you need to condition it into your mind. Here is how to accomplish that:

1. Sit down in a chair. Sit up straight, hands on your lap. Breathe in and out several times.
2. Tell your head to relax, then your eyelids, then your arms and then your legs.
3. Do step number 2 three times very slowly.
4. Think about the picture you admire and see yourself having that physique.
5. SEE yourself moving through the day with that body. SEE others looking at you.
6. HEAR yourself and other people talking to you, notice how you FEEL-notice how they respond to you.
7. FEEL what it would be like to have a body like that. FEEL the emotions you would experience. It could be excitement you feel, or confidence, power, security, attractiveness or something else.

If you notice you don't like what you SEE, HEAR, or FEEL while you are doing this exercise it means: A) you have the wrong picture for you, or B) you have a conflict within yourself (a belief about who you are, what you should be like or how people will respond to you, for example) that needs to be addressed by a professional hypnotherapist.

If you like the sensations you get when you do the conditioning strategy, keep doing it everyday. Make sure you are taking the action steps necessary to achieve this image. Those action steps involve eating right and exercising properly. Condition your mind and your body. Perform your rituals. Rituals are the actions, often very small actions, that lead you to the big actions you want to take. For example, packing your clothes into a gym bag before you leave to workout. Stretching specific body parts before you start your run or powerwalk. One ritual leads to the next and the next until you have performed the behavior you wanted to perform, be it preparing juices or working out. Athletes have many ritualistic behaviors that help them perform well. For example, a baseball pitcher will often look at the catcher, get the signal, look at first base, lift his arms overhead, look at second base, lift his leg, and whip his arm and throw the pitch. These are small rituals, done back-to-back, that lead up to one successful pitch.

We are only touching on hypnosis here. Hypnosis is something to be experienced rather than read about. The subconscious mind is a very powerful force. Get that force working for you and you will achieve your goals and you will enjoy the process more than ever. Let's go now to the next chapter. It is there that you will be given a formula that will systematically change how you look, feel and live. Imagine making a small commitment to...

Chapter 12

Lose 20 lbs. in 30 Days Health Program

"Strength doesn't come from physical capacity. It comes from an individual will"
— Mahatma Gandhi

In order to make this or any program work you must start with your attitude. In other words, the thoughts that you think most often will generate feelings within you and that will eventually direct your actions. Therefore, we will start by understanding our thoughts and changing them so that they support us in reaching our goals. Even if you're on one of those "liquid chocolate" diets you can get results if you are motivated enough. The problem is that sooner or later the negative health effects will become evident and you will have to take steps to reverse them.

This program is healthy and natural. Most people are actually afraid of natural things because we have been conditioned to believe that processed foods and synthetic drugs are the answers to health. These misconceptions are what cause two out of three Americans to be overweight and headed toward serious ill-health conditions. Realize that this program is a healthy life-style approach.

Let's start with your attitude. Why do you want to lose this weight, get in shape, or change your body? How will you feel about yourself? Will you feel that you are achieving what you always dreamed of with your body? Will you feel safer by having muscles or endurance? Will you look better than your ex's new found romance? Write out the benefits that you want to achieve. Make them related to the emotional satisfaction that you will get by accomplishing the goal. Your feelings direct your actions. Master your feelings and you will master your actions. I will show you exactly how to recondition your feelings and actions in the mental conditioning section of this chapter.

Are you absolutely committed to doing whatever it takes to achieve this goal. You may need a few days to get your level of commitment up to 100%. If you are only at 80% then hang around people who are 100% committed and see if it rubs off. If it does you'll know it. You will feel an eager excitement and enthusiasm for achieving what you desire even if you aren't sure if you can do it.

You'll have a mild or moderate obsession with your goal. It's not a bad obsession, it just means you really want what you're after and you'll be 10 times more likely to receive it. Now, commit to doing the disciplines necessary for achieving your goal. If you work in a business or go to school you know that achievement takes daily discipline. It is difficult to run a successful business or get A's in school without attending to the skills and tasks - the disciplines - necessary for the achievement. The same is true here. The consistent, daily disciplines must be done. You can't exercise for five hours one time per week. No, it must be an hour a day or whatever your program calls for at the time. Remember, what success author Jim Rohn says, "discipline weighs ounces, regret weighs tons." If you don't put in an ounce of discipline you will likely suffer tons of regret. Write down your disciplines and commit to doing them. The basic key to success is doing your well thought out disciplines on a daily basis. The basis of failure is called neglect. Neglecting to do what could have been done. Procrastination, or putting off the doable activities that would have led to success after a relatively short while. The first key to this program is to get your mindset and attitude ready. Get excited about your goal; identify the disciplines you need to do (I've done that for you); and then take action consistently. Your success will follow. If for some reason it doesn't it simply means you need a different strategy, or more time, but the habits that lead to success and high self-regard will have been formed.

The next crucial part of your program is movement. Here is your strategy in a nutshell. Move twice per day, for example, morning and evening, for 20 - 30 minutes per session or one time per day for 60 - 90 minutes. You will need to do this 5x per week or more. You will do half of this time as cardiovascular training and half as resistance training or moving your muscles against a specific resistance. Your cardiovascular training will consist of walking, jogging, biking or using an indoor cardiovascular exercise machine. If you decide to exercise for 20 minutes you will break it up like this: 16 minutes at an intensity of three or moderate, 3 minutes at an intensity of four or somewhat hard and 1 minute at an intensity of five or hard (80%, 15%, 5%). Review the Borg Scale chart in the beginning of the book and memorize from numbers two - six. For resistance training, that is, using either your body weight, free weights or machines, you will have to decide what you are willing to invest in. You can check out an exercise video from the library. You could join a gym. You could hire a trainer for a limited or on-going amount of time in order to learn how to lift properly. Half of your movement time will be to improve the strength, shape and endurance of your muscles.

The next part of the program are the Training Secrets. Here they are: **1. When you are doing a muscle strengthening exercise** (i.e. leg lifts, squats, push ups, abdominal curls etc.) **do the movements slowly. 2. Stop at the top.** Hold the body part at the end of the motion for a count of one this will force you to contract the muscle fibers without momentum doing the work instead of your muscles. **3. Vary your exercise every week or so.** Not a lot, but change the number of repetitions, the weight, the sets, the speed or the sequence of the exercises. This forces your muscles and nerves to adapt and that's what you want, adaptive changes. **4. Concentrate.** You will get better results when you fully focus your attention on what you are doing and why you are doing it. Don't read or otherwise distract yourself - it makes a big difference. **5. 80/20 rule.** It has been said, 80% of your results come from 20% of your actions. The last two repetitions out of every ten will produce 80% of your exercise results whereas the first 8 will produce only 20% of your results. The reason is associated with the *overload principle.* You *must* do more than before so that your body will have to adapt and get stronger and change from a flabby shaped muscle to a leaner one. Overload, as described by Bill Pearl four-time Mr. Universe and Gary T. Moran, Ph.D., in Getting Stronger, means that you stress the muscle in intensity or duration beyond the demands of previous activity. This is then followed by a rest period during which the muscle rebuilds with greater strength and endurance. The cells are programmed to rebuild stronger so they can handle greater stress the next time. **6. Body part training.** Eventually, split your workout days into A days and B days. On A days do exercises that work your legs, butt, back and abdominals and on B days work your chest/shoulders/arms and abdominals.

You can do your abdominals virtually everyday unless you are sore. If you are sore do them every other day. Joe Weider, the Master Blaster and body building legend, says that a beginner doing resistance training should wait 48 hours between workouts. For example, workout on Monday, Wednesday and Friday. Those who are more advanced need more recovery - up to three to four days of recuperation. I have noticed this with advanced bodybuilders I have worked with. They claim they make more gains in strength and muscle with more rest. There is much research to support these guidelines - use your body as the judge for you.

The next important part of your program is the *Food Plan.* This plan is designed to be healthy, cleansing and ideal for weight control. First of all, you need to have a good multivitamin-mineral supplement. One that gives at least 100% of the RDA and hopefully more. If you refuse to get one the program will likely still work, but it's not guaranteed. Take 1,500 mg of spirulina. Take 3,000 mg. of vitamin C. Take B complex and B6 and B12 vitamins 50mg. 3x per day. Any other supplements listed in the book will also be beneficial for you. Here is a program that will take the weight off and taste good too.

Week #1:

> *Breakfast:* one medium honeydew melon (or other variety). One 8-12 ounce glass of distilled water with psyllium. Drink <u>water throughout the day</u> ***everyday***
>
> *Lunch:* one 12 -16 ounce carrot, apple, spinach (parsley, or cucumber juice), raw salad with green vegetables and tomato optional. Rice with black or red beans - about 1/2-3/4 cup OR steamed vegetables with tofu (bean curd) - 1/2-1 plate full.
>
> *Dinner:* one glass of distilled water with psyllium; one 12 - 16 ounce carrot, apple, spinach (same as above) juice; raw salad; and tomato, creamed corn, or lentil soup.

Week #2:

> *Break fast:* one apple, one pear and one banana (or another pear). One 8-12 ounce glass of distilled water with psyllium.
>
> *Lunch:* 12 -16 ounces of carrot, beet juice; raw salad as above; hummus with corn bread or spelt (not regu-

lar or wheat bread! *some people are sensitive to wheat) OR Rice with steamed vegetables with tofu.

Dinner: 12 -16 ounces of carrot, beet juice; vegetable stir fry with brown or white rice; 8 ounces of organic baby carrots.

Week #3:

Breakfast Watermelon (or other melon in season) OR mixed fruit salad.

Lunch: 12-16 ounces of carrot, apple parsley juice; about 1/2 -1 cup of rice and red beans; OR steamed vegetables with tofu.

Dinner: 16 ounces of baby carrots; 12 ounces of carrot/apple juice; hummus with corn bread or spelt (and if desired a small raw salad).

Week #4:

Breakfast: 2 apples OR other desired fruit in season; and 12 ounces of carrot juice.

Lunch: 2 egg whites, raw salad, 3/4 cup rice and beans and a few ounces of baby carrots OR steamed vegetables with tofu.

Dinner: 8 ounces of distilled water with psyllium; tomato, creamed corn, or lentil soup; and small portion of brown rice.

* You may add some vegetable protein powder to your juices if you find carbohydrates cause you to gain weight easily. Again, remember to drink plenty of water throughout the day, everyday.
* If still hungry at any point during the day be sure that easy fruit snacks are handy, e.g. grapes, apples, bananas, raisins, etc.

At this point change your diet for 7 - 10 days by going back to a modified version of the above program. Realize that this program is not a diet, it is a life-style change. You can modify the foods based on the seasons, your mood or your desired results. The program is very filling. You will not be hungry physiologically, but mentally it may take getting used to for some people. Some clients feel worse at the beginning because they eliminate coffee, wheat, dairy, meat, fish, sugar and junk food. This detoxification of poisons from your body can make a person feel slightly worse. If that happens to you, drink more water to flush out toxins and know you are cleansing your system. Give yourself time. That is what it takes. If this seems too much for you then start with a one day trial. Later you can add other foods back into your diet that you enjoy. However, you may find that you do not crave certain foods any more because you cleansed your system and allowed your body to desensitize itself to specific foods..

Don't ask, "well, could I just have half a cup of coffee etc. etc.", no. If you vary the program by very much at all my experience is that people end up eating what they normally eat with the exception of maybe one item or simply more fruit. Then they complain if results don't happen overnight. You should not allow yourself to feel hungry. Stick to the program or don't do it - you'll save yourself frustration.

The next important key to your success is *Mental Conditioning:* It is very important that you positively reinforce your good habits each day. You do this by clearing your mind and associating to the positive benefits and feelings that achieving your goals will bring you. You will need to do this activity twice per day for only *two minutes* each. Here's how to do it. Sit in a comfortable position. Close your eyes and take 3 deep, slow breaths and allow yourself to relax. Make a picture in your mind of having what you want - of being the kind of person who can have what you want. Enjoy it. Now see yourself doing all that it takes to accomplish your goals. Feel it, internalize it. By seeing yourself working out and eating right you will be preprogramming yourself to act the way you want to when the situation arises. Now, let's go on to the last key to your super success in the health and fitness game: *Time Mastery.*

Since lack of time is what most people claim is stopping them from exercising we should deal with it. First, schedule your workouts into your day just like any other meeting. Do this on Sunday and review it at night before you go to bed. You can visualize yourself doing your workout at that time during your mental conditioning practice. When the appointed time comes don't analyze it, just get up and move. It is also a good idea to plan when you are going to shop or make food you need to take with you to work or wherever you are going. Master time or time will master you. Be the master or accept being the servant. Remember, there is always time for the important things. Once health and fitness becomes a necessity - a must - then you will make time for it. Give up doing things that no longer serve you. Remember how much time the average person spends in front of the television. Invest 60 minutes of your television time in your health and fitness plan. You mean you don't have a health and fitness plan! Well, now you do. Decide to invest time into your health and fitness plan by setting goals for yourself and acting on them everyday. Instead of trying to fit fitness into your schedule, eliminate things that are wasting your time and your fife.

Identify your priorities - the results you absolutely want to have. Make time for the necessary activities you must do to achieve those results.

Our time together is coming to a close. I hope that you have learned some concepts that will improve your life. Most of all I hope you use what you have read to make changes in yourself for the better and influence those you care about. One last tip: When you see people who are thin, beautiful, fit, shapely or muscular be careful to avoid mocking them. Instead, choose to admire them for their achievement. Because you can not feel good about yourself if you make other people feel bad or put them down. You are not going to achieve something you keep mocking or belittling. Recognize them and think to yourself, "wow, if s/he can do it I can do it too!" One of the greatest things you can do inside or outside a gym is to ask someone who is really fit how they do it and if they can give you a pointer. They will almost always be very happy and flattered to give you free advice. It may differ with what you are reading here, but listen anyway - it will get you enthusiastic about achieving your goals!

Write out your physical fitness goals for the next year by starting one year from now and working backwards. Break them down into monthly, weekly and daily goals for exercise and eating. Remember to include the benefits you will receive for your efforts. Choose activities and foods that you enjoy or will learn to enjoy. If you can learn to enjoy smoking or drinking you can learn to enjoy anything! I hope to see you at one of our seminars or in my travels around the country because I want to tell your successful story to everyone. You can write me, I would really enjoy hearing how you used the strategies and what worked best for you.

The Optimal Performance Institute
520 South Murphy Avenue Ste. 256
Sunnyvale, CA 94086
Attn: John Farley

I wish you all the success in the world, because your health is so important to you and those who care about you - why not start getting healthy and fit today, just like our…

Chapter 13

Case Study

**"To lose patience is
to lose the battle."**
— *Mahatma Gandhi*

Upon reading this book my wife, Janet, decided we needed to have a case study in order to prove what I have been saying throughout the book is true and would work for the average person. I thought about using one of my former clients. While all my clients who stuck with me and did any portion of the **Living Lean!** system improved tremendously, none of them had ever used all of the strategies consistently enough to do a case study on. Besides, we knew that having someone say, "yeah, I used the **Living Lean!** system and it worked!" would not have been enough to convince you that the system can and will work. We wanted to be able to record everything that was happening to the client; all the food eaten, all the exercise completed, even the moods and emotions felt during the entire process. That's when Janet volunteered. Regardless of the results with Janet - individual results vary.

Janet is 29 years old. Though she is a vegetarian for 8 years now, she has always had to struggle with her weight. At 5'4" tall with a medium frame, Janet currently weighs 130 lbs. At her heaviest she weighed 155 lbs. and lightest 115 lbs. It should be noted that Janet had gained 30 lbs. during her freshman year in college and lost it by graduation, three and a half years later, through a running program. She has always had a disproportionate amount of fat on her hips, buttocks and thighs. As an adult, this fat appears as cellulite.

Janet's current fitness level is moderate, she likes to jog occasionally and lift weights when/if she gets to a gym. Her current body fat is 26%. Of her 130 lbs. 34 lbs. are comprised of fat and 96 lbs. comprised of lean mass. Her waist measured in at 30.25 inches, buttocks at 39 inches, thighs at 22 inches and arms at 10.5 inches. Janet's program goals are to lose 10 - 15 lbs., reduce overall bodyfat, shape the gluteal (buttocks) muscles, increase energy, detoxify the body, increase overall musculature and strength, and reduce inches specifically in the buttocks, legs and waist.

I designed the following exercise and nutrition program using the **Living Lean!** system for her based on her goals, and we recorded all the important data over a 34 day period.

In the following pages you will see how one person used the strategies in this book to get in the best shape of her life physically and mentally - so far!

Janet's Living Lean! Program

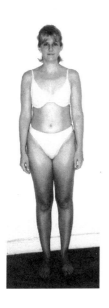

Before the
Living Lean!
program.

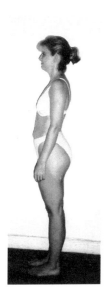

Cardiovascular Training:

40 minutes 2X per day, 7 days per week.
    32 minutes at a level 3/moderate
        intensity
    6 minutes at a level 4/somewhat
        hard intensity
    2 minutes at a level 5/hard
        intensity
Can be powerwalking, jogging, cycling, or
other CV machine.

Weight Training:

Bench press, 8-12 repetitions, 3 sets
Lat pulldown, 8-12 repetitions, 3 sets
Seated row, 8-12 repetitions, 3 sets
Lateral raises, 8-12 repetitions, 3 sets
Bicep curls, 8-12 repetitions, 3 sets
Tricep pushdowns, 8-12 repetitions, 3 sets
One legged squats, 10X each, 2 sets
Smith squats, 8-12 repetitions, 3 sets
Leg extension, 8-12 repetitions, 3 sets
Leg raises, 10 repetitions, 3 sets - hold
    for 10 secs. at top.
Abdominals, 25 crunches, 25 X-overs
    each side.
Back extension, 10 repetitions, 2 sets
Stretches

Mental Conditioning:

Hypnosis session 1X at the beginning of
the program.

Supplements:

Taken daily, throughout the day;

Spirulina	one tablet
Vit C	4,000 mg.
L-carnitine	one tablet
B complex (B6, B12)	one tablet
Vit E	400 IU
Chromium	400 mcg.
multi/Nutra Source	one tablet
Pycnogenol	one tablet
CoEnzyme Q10	60 mg.
Vegetable protein powder	

Nutrition:

Breakfast
Eat 1-2 cups of mellon or seasonal fruit
Lunch
Have a rice, bean, tofu and/or vegetable mixture for lunch.
Dinner
Have fruit salad or single fruits and throughout the evening if necessary.

Daily
Drink 8-16 ounces of carrot/apple/spinach or lettuce juice every 3 hours (minumum of 32 ounces per day).

Avoid wheat and gluten products.

Consume a minimum of 50 grams of proten per day.

Drink an additional 32 ounces of distilled water daily.

Special
Vegetable juice and whole fruit fast on **Sundays**.

Exercise and Food log for Janet

Day 1 Friday
130lbs/BF%=26/w=30.25"/b=39"/t=22"

40min on StairMaster at level 3 (8:30am)
40min jog on treadmill 5mph (4pm)
weight program (light weights)
                    Took all vitamins listed throughout the day
9:30am - bowl of watermelon
12noon - 16oz carrot/apple/spinach juice
2pm - steamed vegetables w/ brown rice
4pm - banana
6:15pm - 16oz carrot juice
6:30pm - bowl of watermelon
9:30pm - small bowl of watermelon

NOTE: I felt very motivated, and was not hungry at all.

Day 2   Saturday

40min on StairMaster at level 3 (8:30am)
40min powerwalk - brisk pace (5pm)
                    Took all vitamins listed throughout the day
10:45am - bowl of watermelon
12:15pm - 16oz carrot/pear/spinach juice
1:45pm - Luna® Bar
3:45pm - steamed vegetables w/ brown rice
7pm - 16oz carrot juice
7:15pm - bowl of cherries
8:30pm - 16oz carrot/pear/spinach juice

NOTE: I felt a little tired today, but still motivated. Again I was not hungry at all, in fact I felt 'overful'.

Day 3   Sunday

40min on StairMaster at level 3 (9:30am)

40min powerwalk - brisk pace (6pm)
Took all vitamins listed throughout the day
10:30am - bowl of watermelon
12:30pm - 16oz carrot/apple juice
2:45pm - bowl watermelon
3pm - apple juice w/ protein powder
6pm - 16oz carrot/apple juice
6:30pm - bowl of cherries
8:30pm - "Fresh Samantha" Berry juice

NOTE: I felt very, very energized today, and was not hungry at all.

Day 4   Monday
40min on StairMaster at level 3 (9:00am)
40min jog on treadmill 5mph (5pm)
weight program (light weights)
Took all vitamins listed throughout the day
10:30am - bowl of watermelon
11:30am - Luna® Bar
12noon - 16oz carrot juice
1pm - Medium black bean burrito
2:30pm - "Fresh Samantha" Raspberry juice
6:00pm - 16oz carrot/apple juice
6:30pm - small bowl of watermelon
7:00pm - "Fresh Samantha" Cranberry juice

NOTE: I felt good, working hard.

Day 5   Tuesday
40min on StairMaster at level 3 (8:30am)
40min powerwalk - brisk pace (5pm)
Took all vitamins listed throughout the day
12noon - bowl of watermelon
12:30pm - Luna® Bar
2pm - Medium black bean burrito
2:30pm - "Fresh Samantha" juice

5pm - 16oz carrot/apple juice
7:45pm - 16oz carrot juice
8:00pm - large pear

NOTE: I felt very motivated, and was not very hungry today.

Day 6   Wednesday

40min on StairMaster at level 3 (8:30am)
40min jog on treadmill 5.2mph (5pm)
weight program (light-medium weights)
                Took all vitamins listed throughout the day
10:00am - bowl of watermelon
11:00am - Luna® Bar
12:45pm - 16oz carrot/apple juice
1:15pm - Medium black bean burrito
6:00pm - 16oz carrot/apple juice
6:45pm - large banana
8:00pm - "Fresh Samantha" juice

NOTE: I felt very strong and motivated.

Day 7   Thursday

40min on StairMaster at level 3 (8:30am)
40min powerwalk - brisk pace (4pm)
                Took all vitamins listed throughout the day
10:00am - medium banana
10:30am - medium banana
1:00pm - 16oz carrot/apple juice
2:30pm - 1/2 box Goya® black beans & rice
5:30pm - Luna® Bar
7:30pm - bowl of cherries
8:30pm - "Fresh Samantha" juice

NOTE: I felt a bit sluggish today, but I'm getting into a groove.

Day 8   Friday

128lbs/BF%=25.3/w=28.87"/b=38.87"/t=22.37"

40min on StairMaster at level 3-4 (8:30am)
40min jog on treadmill 5.2mph (4pm)
weight program (light-medium weights)
     Took all vitamins listed throughout the day
10:30am - bowl of cherries
12:30pm - 16oz carrot/apple/spinach juice
2:45pm - Luna® Bar
5:45pm - 16oz carrot/apple juice
6:30pm - bowl of cherries
8:30pm - cranberry juice w/ protein powder

NOTE: I felt a bit frustrated today, all this hard work and I only lost 2lbs.

Day 9 Saturday

40min powerwalk - brisk pace (10:30am)
40min powerwalk - brisk pace (6pm)
     Took all vitamins listed throughout the day
12:30pm - 16oz carrot/apple juice
1:00pm - 3 egg whites
2:30pm - 1/2 box Goya® black beans & rice
5:30pm - 16oz carrot juice
7:30pm - bowl of cherries
8:30pm - "Fresh Samantha" juice

NOTE: I felt energized and remotivated.

Day 10 Sunday

40min powerwalk - brisk pace (11:00am)
40min powerwalk - brisk pace (6pm)
     Took all vitamins listed throughout the day
12noon - large banana
1:15pm - 16oz carrot/apple juice
1:45pm - large banana

5:45pm - bowl of watermelon
7:15pm - 16oz carrot/apple juice
8:15pm - large peach
8:30pm - "Fresh Samantha" juice

NOTE: I felt even more motivated, I weighed myself again and lost 2 more pounds.

Day 11   Monday

40min on StairMaster at level 4-5 (8:30am)
40min jog on treadmill 5.3mph (4pm)
weight program (medium weights)
                Took all vitamins listed throughout the day
10:45am - large peach
12:30pm - 1/2 box Goya® red beans & rice
4:15pm - 16oz carrot/lettuce juice
7:00pm - bowl of cherries
8:15pm - 16oz carrot/lettuce juice

NOTE: I felt good and strong today, very motivated as a result of yesterdays weigh-in. I was not very hungry.

Day 12   Tuesday

40min on StairMaster at level 4-5 (8:30am)
40min powerwalk - brisk pace (5pm)
                Took all vitamins listed throughout the day
10:45am - bowl of watermelon
12:15pm - 16oz carrot/apple juice
1:00pm - protein drink
1:30pm - 1/2 box Goya® black beans & rice
4:15pm - "Fresh Samantha" juice
7:15pm - 16oz carrot/lettuce juice
8:00pm - large peach

NOTE: I felt great today!

Day 13   Wednesday

40min on StairMaster at level 4-6 (8:30am)
40min jog on treadmill 5.5mph (5pm)
weight program (medium-heavy weights)
            Took all vitamins listed throughout the day
12noon - vegetables w/ rice
1:30pm - 16oz carrot/apple/spinach juice
4:30pm -large banana
6:30pm - protein drink
8:30pm - 16oz carrot/apple juice
9:30pm - bowl of cherries

NOTE: I felt great!

Day 14   Thursday
124lbs/BF%=24.6/w=28.25/b=38.5/t=22.37

40min on StairMaster at level 3 (8:30am)
            Took all vitamins listed throughout the day
10:00am - large bowl of watermelon
11:00am - 16oz carrot/apple juice
12:30pm -Luna® Bar
5:00pm - protein drink
6:00pm - "Fresh Samantha"
7:00pm - spaghetti w/ oil & garlic & bread

NOTE: I felt good. Went on a trip out of town.

Day 15   Friday

40min jog outside (7:30pm)
            Took all vitamins listed throughout the day
10:00am - "Fresh Samantha" juice
11:00am - 2 oranges
2:00pm - large salad w/ portabello mushroom
6:15pm - apple juice

8:30pm - 16oz carrot/apple juice
6:45pm - peach

NOTE: I felt very strong and motivated.

Day 16   Saturday

40min on StairMaster at level 4-5 (10:30am)
40min jog on treadmill 5.2mph (5pm)
weight program (medium weights)
                    Took all vitamins listed throughout the day
10:00am - bowl of watermelon
11am - Luna® Bar
12:45pm -16oz carrot/apple juice
1:15pm - 1/2 box Goya® black beans & rice
6:00pm - 16oz carrot/apple juice
6:45pm - large banana
8:00pm - "Fresh Samantha" juice

NOTE: I felt very strong and motivated.

Day 17   Sunday

40min powerwalk - brisk pace (11:30am)
40min powerwalk - brisk pace (4pm)
                    Took all vitamins listed throughout the day
12noon - bowl of watermelon
1:00pm - protein drink
2:45pm -16oz carrot/apple juice
6:00pm - 16oz carrot/apple juice
6:45pm - large banana
8:00pm - "Fresh Samantha" juice

NOTE: I felt very good.

Day 18   Monday

40min on StairMaster at level 3 (8:30am)

40min jog outside (6pm)
weight program (heavy weights)
                Took all vitamins listed throughout the day
10:00am - large banana
12noon - vegetables w/ rice & tofu
2:30pm -banana
3:00pm - 16oz carrot/apple juice
6:30pm - protein drink
7:00pm - 16oz carrot/spinach juice
8:00pm - Luna® Bar

NOTE: I felt great and my run was awesome!!

Day 19   Tuesday
40min on StairMaster at level 4-6 (8:30am)
40min jog outside (6pm)
                Took all vitamins listed throughout the day
10:00am - 16oz carrot/apple/spinach juice
11:00am - large apricot
12:30pm -vegetables w/ rice-noodles & tofu
3:15pm - 16oz carrot/apple juice
6:00pm - protein drink
6:45pm - large banana
8:00pm - "Fresh Samantha" juice

NOTE: I felt very strong and motivated.

Day 20   Wednesday
40min on StairMaster at level 4-6 (8:30am)
40min jog on treadmill 5.6mph (5pm)
weight program (heavy weights)
                Took all vitamins listed throughout the day
9:30am - large plum
11:00am - 16oz carrot juice
11:30pm - 2 egg whites
12:00pm - 2 egg whites w/ vegetables & rice

6:00pm - protein drink
6:45pm - large plum
8:00pm - 16oz carrot/apple juice

NOTE: I felt great!

Day 21   Thursday
40min on StairMaster at level 4-6 (8:30am)
40min powerwalk - brisk pace (6pm)
　　　　　Took all vitamins listed throughout the day
10:00am - large apricot
11:00am - 16oz carrot/apple juice
12:00pm - protein drink
1:15pm - vegetables w/ rice & tofu
6:00pm - 16oz carrot/apple juice
8:00pm - "Fresh Samantha" juice

NOTE: I felt good.

Day 22   Friday
121lbs/BF%=20.8/w=27"/b=37.87"/t=22"
40min on StairMaster at level 4-6 (8:30am)
40min jog on treadmill 5.6mph (5pm)
weight program (heavy weights)
　　　　　Took all vitamins listed throughout the day
11:00am - protein drink
1:30pm - tofu w/ beans
2:45pm -16oz carrot/apple juice
3:15pm - 16oz carrot/apple/spinach juice
4:00pm - 2 large plums
6:45pm - protein drink
8:00pm - "Fresh Samantha" juice

NOTE: I felt very awesome mentally, but very tired, I have my
period.

Day 23   Saturday

40min powerwalk - brisk pace (10:30am)
40min jog outside (5pm)
       Took all vitamins listed throughout the day
12noon - "Fresh Samantha" juice
12:30pm - Luna® Bar
1:45pm -16oz carrot/apple juice
2:15pm - vegetable w/ rice & tofu
6:00pm - 16oz carrot/apple juice
6:45pm - protein drink
8:00pm - "Fresh Samantha" juice

NOTE: I felt all right today, but not spectacular.

Day 24   Sunday

40min powerwalk - brisk pace (11:30am)
40min powerwalk - brisk pace (5pm)
       Took all vitamins listed throughout the day
12noon - bowl of watermelon
1:00pm - "Fresh Samantha" juice
2:45pm -16oz carrot/apple juice
6:00pm - 16oz carrot/apple juice
6:45pm - large banana
8:00pm - "Fresh Samantha" juice

NOTE: I felt stronger today.

Day 25   Monday

40min on StairMaster at level 4-6 (8:30am)
40min jog on treadmill 5.8mph (5pm)
weight program (heavy weights)
       Took all vitamins listed throughout the day
10:00am - large plum
11:15am - Luna® Bar
12:45pm -16oz carrot/apple juice
1:15pm - vegetables w/ rice & tofu

6:00pm - 16oz carrot/apple juice
6:45pm - large plum
8:00pm - "Fresh Samantha" juice

NOTE: I felt great!

Day 26   Tuesday

40min on StairMaster at level 4-6 (8:30am)
40min jog outside (6pm)
> Took all vitamins listed throughout the day

10:00am - large plum
11:00am - Luna® Bar
12noon - 2 egg whites
12:45pm -16oz carrot/apple juice
1:15pm - vegetables w/ rice & tofu
6:00pm - 16oz carrot/apple juice
6:45pm - Luna® Bar
8:00pm - "Fresh Samantha" juice

NOTE: I felt very strong and motivated.

Day 27   Wednesday

40min on StairMaster at level 4-6 (8:30am)
40min jog on treadmill 5.8mph (5pm)
weight program (heavy weights)
> Took all vitamins listed throughout the day

10:00am - large plum
11:15am - Luna® Bar
12:30pm -16oz carrot/apple/spinach juice
1:15pm - vegetables w/ rice & tofu
3:00pm - 2 egg whites
6:00pm - 16oz carrot/apple juice
8:00pm - "Fresh Samantha" juice

NOTE: I felt very good.

Day 28   Thursday

40min on StairMaster at level 3 (8:30am)
40min jog on treadmill 5.2mph (5pm)
        Took all vitamins listed throughout the day
10:00am - large plum
11:30am - Luna® Bar
12:45pm -16oz carrot/apple juice
1:45pm - vegetables w/ rice & tofu
6:00pm - 16oz carrot/apple juice
6:30pm - Luna® Bar
8:15pm - "Fresh Samantha" juice

NOTE: I felt thin!!!!

Day 29   Friday

40min on StairMaster at level 4-6 (8:30am)
40min jog on treadmill 5.8mph (5pm)
weight program (heavy weights)
        Took all vitamins listed throughout the day
10:00am - large plum
11:00am - Luna® Bar
12:15pm -16oz carrot/apple juice
1:45pm - vegetables w/ rice & tofu
6:00pm - 16oz carrot/apple juice
6:45pm - large plum
8:00pm - "Fresh Samantha" juice

NOTE: I felt awesome!

Day 30   Saturday

40min powerwalk - brisk pace (11:30am)
40min powerwalk - brisk pace (6pm)
        Took all vitamins listed throughout the day
1:00pm - large bowl of watermelon
2:00pm - 16oz carrot/apple/spinach juice
4:00pm - large bowl watermelon

6:45pm - protein drink
8:00pm - 16oz carrot/apple/spinach juice

NOTE: I felt awesome!

Day 31   Sunday

40min powerwalk - brisk pace (11:45am)
40min powerwalk - brisk pace (6pm)
    Took all vitamins listed throughout the day
12noon - bowl of watermelon
1:30pm - "Fresh Samantha" juice
2:45pm -16oz carrot/apple juice
5:00pm - 16oz carrot/apple juice
6:30pm - large peach
8:00pm - "Fresh Samantha" juice

NOTE: I felt great today.

Day 32   Monday

40min on StairMaster at level 4-6 (8:00am)
40min jog on treadmill 5.8mph (5pm)
weight program (heavy weights)
    Took all vitamins listed throughout the day
10:00am - large plum
11:00am - Luna® Bar
12:45pm -16oz carrot/apple juice
1:15pm - vegetables w/ rice & tofu
6:00pm - 16oz carrot/apple/spinach juice
6:45pm - large banana
8:00pm - "Fresh Samantha" juice

NOTE: I felt great!

Day 33   Tuesday

40min on StairMaster at level 4-6 (9:00am)
40min jog outside (6pm)

Took all vitamins listed throughout the day

10:30am - large plum
11:15am - Luna® Bar
12noon - 3 egg whites
12:30pm -16oz carrot/apple juice
1:15pm - vegetables w/ rice & tofu
6:00pm - 16oz carrot/apple juice
6:45pm - Luna® Bar
8:00pm - "Fresh Samantha" juice

NOTE: I felt very strong and motivated.

Day 34   Wednesday
118lbs./BF%=19.5/w=26.75"/b=37.5"/t=22"

40min on StairMaster at level 4-6 (8:30am)
40min jog on treadmill 5.8mph (5pm)
weight program (heavy weights)

Took all vitamins listed throughout the day

10:00am - large peach
11:15am - Luna® Bar
12:45pm -16oz carrot/apple/spinach juice
1:45pm - vegetables w/ rice & tofu
3:00pm - 2 egg whites
6:00pm - 16oz carrot/apple juice
8:00pm - "Fresh Samantha" juice

NOTE: I felt very great!!!!.

Drum Roll, Please…

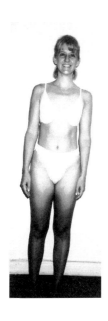

After
Living Lean!
program

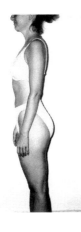

Janet's physiological measurements were taken every week. We used caliper and Futrex 5000 to measure her body fat percentages.

Some weeks her weight would change very little until the end of the week or the beginning of the next week. Some weeks she would lose weight quickly and then taper off quickly. While the measurements give objective numbers by which to judge her progress, there were also many subjective benefits. The less measurable, but equally important changes included: better sleep, more energy, less bagginess under the eyes, changes in the way her muscles and body actually feel, and increased motivation to achieve.

I hypnotized Janet during the first weekend of the program. After a 45 minute session she was motivated to do the program and had vivid images in her mind of what to achieve. After the second week I suggested she add more protein to her diet to allow her body to avoid using her own muscles for fuel. She did add protein and it helped her continue to drop weight and stay energized. She was told to never be hungry. She could always eat anytime she felt the desire, but she was initially too full from the foods on her plan. Each person needs to make their own decisions as to when to eat and when not to.

I suggested she avoid wheat / gluten. The reason was that it has been reported that some people get cellulite due to food sensitivities or allergies. A former client of mine by the name of Donna once lost eight (8) pounds in eight (8) days when I took her off all wheat products. Her medical history showed a mild sensitivity to wheat. She felt miserable for the first three days and then she felt light and energized as the weight came off.

I insisted Janet perform the type of weight exercises and other resistance exercises I designed for her buttocks (gluteal) region. After I coached her on two occasions she started making marked improvements on her buttocks (gluteal) region.

Janet lost an average of 3 pounds each week she was on the program - some weeks four pounds were dropped, other weeks two pounds. She did lose the amount of weight that was comfortable for her while keeping her motivation high enough to continue training until the habits were strengthened. We estimate she still has 5-7 pounds to lose in her buttocks region. Her body is changing physiologically and biochemically. The fat in the buttocks region is disappearing from the 'out-side-in' - from the top and bottom as the changes move toward the middle.

The Tale Of The Tape
After 34 Days

- Decreased weight by 12 pounds

- Decreased 6.5% in body fat

- Decreased 3.5 inches in her waist

- Decreased 2.5 inches in her buttocks

- Maintained thigh size although fluctuations happened throughout the program. Definite changes in the muscle/fat ratio were detected upon palpitation.

- Motivation to continue with the life-style changes in order to reduce another five pounds of body fat while increasing muscle weight by several pounds.

- More energy, better sleep, more motivation, more endurance, happier, feels better.

Keep these points in mind: Your body is different from Janet's and others. Often the more weight a person has to lose the faster the initial reduction. This is not always the case - bodies differ. Janet has never been able to dramatically reduce her gluteal area and now for the first time it appears that she will achieve her goal faster than ever imagined. We will change her routine to concentrate on the buttocks and in a few weeks not only will her weight be lower, but also her trouble spots will disappear! Imagine having a great body in 30 to 60 days - its fantastic.

Now it is your turn. Make the commitment, learn what steps you need to take - they are in this book - and then take them. Make exercise and eating fun and challenging and you will accomplish your health and fitness goals. Good luck and best wishes to you.

Journal Forms

Exercise Record

DATE: _____ / _____ / _____   DAY #: _____

Cardiovascular Training

Warm-up (5 - 10min)		RPE Level		Type of Exercise	
AM	PM	AM	PM	AM	PM
Workout (10 - 60min)		**RPE Level**		**Type of Exercise**	
AM	PM	AM	PM	AM	PM
Cool-down (5 - 10min)		**RPE Level**		**Type of Exercise**	
AM	PM	AM	PM	AM	PM

Resistance Training

Exercise	Weight	Set #1	Set #2	Set #3	Set #4	Set #5
	lbs	reps	reps	reps	reps	reps
	lbs	reps	reps	reps	reps	reps
	lbs	reps	reps	reps	reps	reps
	lbs	reps	reps	reps	reps	reps
	lbs	reps	reps	reps	reps	reps
	lbs	reps	reps	reps	reps	reps
	lbs	reps	reps	reps	reps	reps
	lbs	reps	reps	reps	reps	reps
	lbs	reps	reps	reps	reps	reps
	lbs	reps	reps	reps	reps	reps

Nutrition Record

DATE: _____ / _____ / _____   DAY #: _____

TIME	FOOD INTAKE	CALORIES
_____:_____ AM/PM		
_____:_____ AM/PM		
_____:_____ AM/PM		
_____:_____ AM/PM		
_____:_____ AM/PM		
_____:_____ AM/PM		
_____:_____ AM/PM		
_____:_____ AM/PM		
DAILY TOTAL		

Today I feel: ❑ ENERGETIC ❑ MOTIVATED ❑ HAPPY ❑ SLOW
❑ TIRED ❑ DEPRESSED ❑ OUT OF CONTROL ❑ _____

Exercises

Exercises

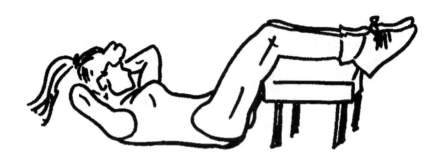

Abdominals: With feet on a chair (90° angle) or on the floor (45° angle), place your hands behind your head or place them on your chest (more difficult). Lift your chest 30° off the floor (bringing your shoulder blades off the floor) 10 - 50 times, 2 - 5 sets. This strengthens and tightens the abdominals as well as lower back.

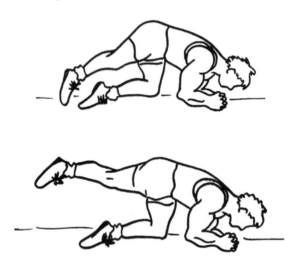

Leg Raises: With elbows and knees on the floor, head in line with the spine, lift one leg slowly just higher than the buttocks 10 - 40 times each leg, 2 - 5 sets. This strengthens and firms the gluteal muscles.

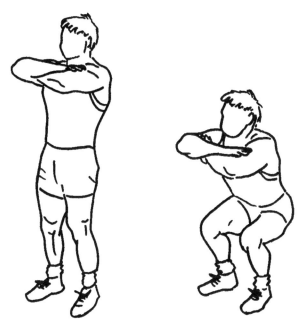

Squats: Hands in front of chest. Feet shoulder width apart. Eyes 45°
in front. Keeping back straight, bend knees until thigh is parallel to
the floor and then return to standing 5 - 20 times, 2 - 5 sets. This
strengthens the quadraceps and gluteals (buttocks).

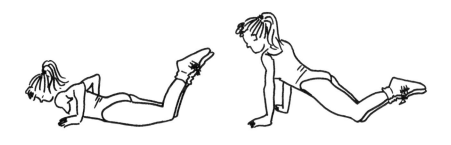

Modified Pushups: With knees on the floor. Hands shoulder width
apart. Back straight. Lift your chest off the floor 2 - 20 times, 2 - 5
sets. This strengthen the chest, triceps and shoulders.

Stretches

Stretches

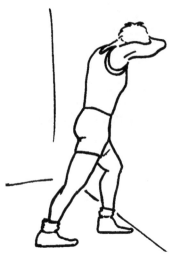

Calf Stretch: Face a wall or chair an arms length away. Lean on the wall, bend the left knee keep the right knee straight pushing your heal into the floor. Hold for 20 - 60 seconds, switch legs. This stretches the gastrocnemius muscle.

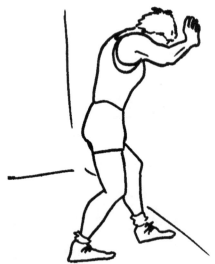

Deep Calf Stretch: Face a wall or chair an arms length away. Lean on the wall, bend the left knee, bend the right knee and sit back to stretch the muscle. Hold for 20 - 60 seconds, switch legs. This stretches the soleus muscle.

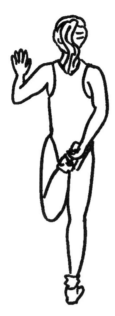

Quad Stretch: While holding on to something, grab your foot and bring it to your buttocks. Keep the bent knee close to the straight leg. Hold for 20 - 60 seconds, switch legs. This stretches your quadriceps muscles.

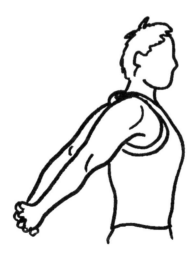

Shoulder Stretch: Clasp your hands behind your back and raise them towards the sky. Hold for 20 - 60 seconds. This stretches your anterior deltoids.

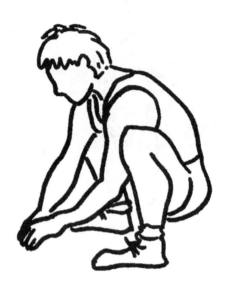

Low back Stretch: Squat down, feet flat on the floor. Hug your legs for balance. Hold for 20 - 60 seconds. This stretches the lower back muscles.

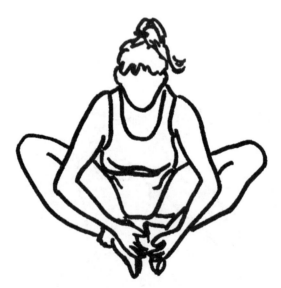

Inner Thigh Stretch: Sit on the floor, bring your knees toward you, bottoms of feet together. Press your knees toward the floor. Hold for 20 - 60 seconds. This stretches your inner thigh muscles.

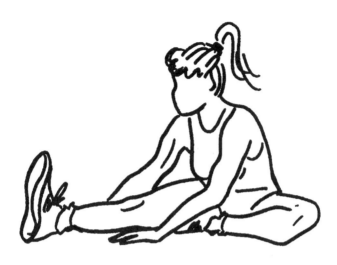

Hamstring Stretch: Sit on the floor. With one leg our straight and one bent inward, lean forward, back straight. Attempt to touch your far toe. Hold for 20 - 60 seconds. This stretches the hamstring muscles.

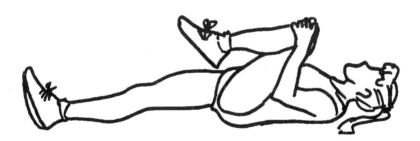

Back and Buttock Stretch: Lie on your back. Pull one leg toward your chest, keeping the other leg straight. Exhale and relax. Hold for 20 - 60 seconds. This stretches the low back and gluteal muscles.

✎ **NOTES:**

✎   **NOTES:**

✍   **NOTES:**

About The Author

John Farley, MA, has traveled the country sharing fitness, nutrition, and motivation/sports psychology seminars providing information to various groups of people. He has been on Good Morning America Sunday, Japanese Television, and Long Island Television programs and has been featured in Self magazine, The Chicago Tribune, The Village Voice, HealthMap, New York Bodies, and local newspapers.

John Farley is the president of The Optimal Performance Institute (OPI) a nonprofit educational institution. Mr. Farley oversees OPI's Sports Psychology Certification and Degree programs, as well as, the Business Communications program. He has his Masters degree from Teachers College, Columbia University in Exercise Science, as well as hypnosis and Neuro-Linguistic Programming certificates. John is a former regional and national karate champion. He is available for a limited number of speaking engagements each year on stress management and healthy living.

For a catalog from The Optimal Performance Institute
Visit our website at www.opi-university.org

John Farley's
PowerWalking! System

30 Minutes Each Side
$15.00

Side A: John Farley personally coaches you to get and
stay motivated to the inspirational and upbeat instru-
mental music. Plus, John
challenges you with 5 one-
minute intervals to boost
your metabolism and burn
more calories.

Side B: Music only! The in-
strumental sounds of ca-
lypso, rock & roll, marches
and more will keep you motivated as you burn fat and
become energized.

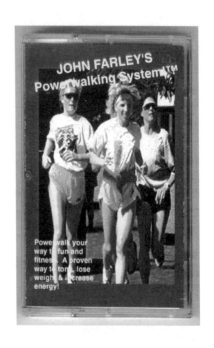

This program features a warm-up and cool-down period, and is approximately **60 minutes** in length. Aerobic interval training, as featured in the program, is scientifically proven to increase cardiovascular endurance more effectively than ordinary steady state aerobic
exercise. Rate of Perceived Exertion (RPE) scale included.

To order, see form in back of book
or call **1-800-607-0369**
or visit our website at **www.LivingLean.org**

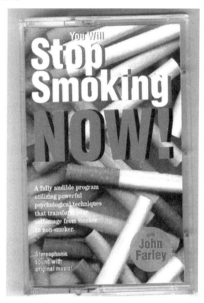

Supplements

Nutra Trim Weight Loss Supplement
$11.95
Diet Booster with Chromium Picolinate
90 Tablets (30 day supply)

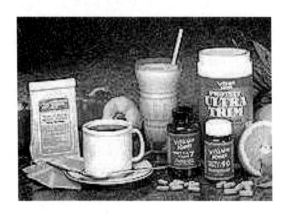

Chromium Picolinate	200 mcg
Herbal Complex (Cornsilk, Parsley, Uva Ursi)	600 mg
Phenylalanine	100 mg
Kelp	100 mg
Soya Lecithin	1200 mg
Vitamin B-6 (Pyridoxine HCL)	50 mg
Cider Vinegar	240 mg

In a natural nutritious base containing Oat Bran Fiber, Parsley, Watercress, Psyllium, and Wheat Germ
Other ingredients: dicalcium phosphate, microcrystalline cellulose, stearic acid, silica, croscarmellose sodium, magnesium stearate and pharmaceutical glaze. This product is formulated without added sugar, starch, salt, corn, wheat, artificial coloring, flavoring or preservatives.

Supplements

Nutra Source 100
$23.95
Over 100 Food Source Nutrients per Tablet, No Iron Added!
180 Tablets (60 day supply)

Super Phyto-Nutrients, Multi-Vitamins, Chelated Minerals,
Digestive Enzymes, Anti-Oxidants, Bioflavonoids, Herbs…

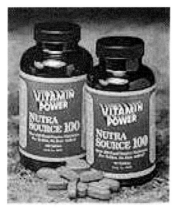

Nutra Source 100 - A total wellness, super multi-nutrient formula from the earth's riches sources… Vitamin Power's new Nutra Source 100 tablets supply protective Phyto-Nutrients including Carotenoids, Flavonoids, and Phytosterols plus Multi-Vitamins, Chelated Minerals (without Iron!), Digestive Enzymes, Anti Oxidants, Bioflavonoids, Herbs… over 100 whole food nutrients all-in-one formula. Extensive media attention has increased awareness about the important health benefits of protective Phyto-Nutrients. These powerful, natural food factors are active plant constituents from fruit, green foods, soy, grains, cruciferous vegetables and herbs. Naturally energized from rays of the sun, Phyto-Nutrients provide maximum protection against free radicals while building a strong immune system. Nutra-Source 100 is a powerful multi-nutrient formula supplying maximum potency for optimum nutritional performance.

It's the next step beyond multivitamins!

John Farley's
E-FitnessTrainer Program
Based on the Living Lean! System

Now, you can work with John Farley and his certified personal fitness trainers directly, no matter where you are in the world - even when you travel. The program is a revolutionary method based on the Living Lean! weight management and lifestyle program. If you ever wanted to get in the best shape of your life and feel better, now you really can.

The E-FitnessTrainer system is like no other in the world. You have a personal relationship with your trainer and John Farley 5 days per week. John and your trainer know your name and what your needs and goals are. Your fitness and nutritional plans are prepared for you based on the information you supply. Each day, Monday - Friday, you e-mail your trainer with your training log form. Your trainer and John Farley review the form and email you back with educational and motivational information and insights that insure your workout and nutritional plan are effective.

You receive everything you need in order to jump start your healthy, lean lifestyle. Included in your program are:
- Supplements required for detoxification, fat reduction, muscular enhancement, and general good health. ($300 value)
- Your own personally designed fitness plan based on your goals.
- Your own personally designed nutritional plan based on your goals.
- Access to John Farley and your trainer Monday - Friday.
- Total flexibility to work out when and where you choose.
- Motivation, counseling, education, advice, support, direction, results.

The total *E-FitnessTrainer Program with John Farley* is **only $599.95** for 6 weeks.

Remember, you receive: <u>$300 worth of necessary dietary supplements and access to John Farley and your own personal trainer Monday - Friday for</u> **6 full weeks.**

     Supplements will last each person from 2 - 6 months. Your program will jump start your attitude, mood and results. From then on, you'll be able to live your life better, look better, feel better and accomplish all the other important things you want to achieve with your new found energy and confidence.

     As you can imagine, this program is very limited and exclusive. People are joining and finishing the program all the time. Now is your chance to make a change for the better. Don't let this moment slip by without taking action. Go to our website today and learn the weight management system that will revolutionize your life!

To enroll,
call **1-800-607-0369**
or visit our website at **www.LivingLean.org**

John Farley's
On-Line
Weight Management
Club

For more information visit our website at...

www.LivingLean.org

Audio Cassettes
with John Farley, M.A.

Super Nutrition I

This audio tape explores nutrition for those who want to get healthy and lose weight. Foods to consume and foods to avoid and why.

Super Nutrition II

This program picks up where Super Nutrition I left off. More keys to eating and drinking your way to health, energy and weight control.

Reverse Aging I

The concept of aging is taught and the basics of how to reverse it. A must for those who want to remain youthful.

Reverse Aging II

A continuation of how to reverse aging and remain youthful. Increase energy, improve physiological functioning and bring your body and mind back to when you were younger and stronger.

Mastering Stress

This audiocassette program will teach you how you respond to the stress impacting you, each day. You will learn how to identify your stressors and de-stress your life.

Order Form

Please send me the following products & programs:

		Price	Quantity	TOTAL
❑	**PowerWalking!** System	$ 15.00	X _____	_____
❑	You will **Stop Smoking Now!**	$ 19.95	X _____	_____
❑	Nutra Trim	$ 11.95	X _____	_____
❑	Nutra Source 100	$ 23.95	X _____	_____
❑	**Living Lean!** Journal	$ 9.95	X _____	_____

Additional audiocassettes by John Farley:

		Price	Quantity	TOTAL
❑	Super Nutrition I	$ 9.95*	X _____	_____
❑	Super Nutrition II	$ 9.95*	X _____	_____
❑	Reverse Aging I	$ 9.95*	X _____	_____
❑	Reverse Aging II	$ 9.95*	X _____	_____
❑	Mastering Stress	$ 9.95*	X _____	_____

* Purchase any four (4) tapes and get the fifth tape FREE!

TOTAL: _____

S&H: **$3.50**

AMOUNT ENCLOSED: _____

❑ Check/Cash   ❑ Visa/MasterCard   ❑ Amercian Express

Card # _____ Exp. _____

Signature _____ Date _____

Name _____

Address _____

City _____ State _____ Zip _____

Phone number (____) _____ — _____

To order simply tear out the order form and mail it to
The Optimal Performance Institute
520 S. Murphy Ave. Ste. 256, Sunnyvale, CA 94086
or call **1-800-607-0369**
or visit our website at **www.LivingLean.org**

Order Form

Please send me the following products & programs:

		Price	Quantity	TOTAL
❏	**PowerWalking!** System	$ 15.00	X _____	_____
❏	You will **Stop Smoking Now!**	$ 19.95	X _____	_____
❏	Nutra Trim	$ 11.95	X _____	_____
❏	Nutra Source 100	$ 23.95	X _____	_____
❏	**Living Lean!** Journal	$ 9.95	X _____	_____

Additional audiocassettes by John Farley:

		Price	Quantity	TOTAL
❏	Super Nutrition I	$ 9.95*	X _____	_____
❏	Super Nutrition II	$ 9.95*	X _____	_____
❏	Reverse Aging I	$ 9.95*	X _____	_____
❏	Reverse Aging II	$ 9.95*	X _____	_____
❏	Mastering Stress	$ 9.95*	X _____	_____

* Purchase any four (4) tapes and get the fifth tape FREE!

TOTAL: _____

S&H: **$3.50**

AMOUNT ENCLOSED: _____

❏ Check/Cash   ❏ Visa/MasterCard   ❏ Amercian Express

Card # _____   Exp. _____

Signature _____   Date _____

Name _____

Address _____

City _____ State _____ Zip _____

Phone number (   ) _____ — _____

To order simply tear out the order form and mail it to
The Optimal Performance Institute
520 S. Murphy Ave. Ste. 256, Sunnyvale, CA 94086
or call **1-800-607-0369**
or visit our website at **www.LivingLean.org**

Order Form

Please send me the following products & programs:

		Price	Quantity	TOTAL
❑	**PowerWalking!** System	$ 15.00	X _____	_____
❑	You will **Stop Smoking Now!**	$ 19.95	X _____	_____
❑	Nutra Trim	$ 11.95	X _____	_____
❑	Nutra Source 100	$ 23.95	X _____	_____
❑	**Living Lean!** Journal	$ 9.95	X _____	_____

Additional audiocassettes by John Farley:

		Price	Quantity	TOTAL
❑	Super Nutrition I	$ 9.95*	X _____	_____
❑	Super Nutrition II	$ 9.95*	X _____	_____
❑	Reverse Aging I	$ 9.95*	X _____	_____
❑	Reverse Aging II	$ 9.95*	X _____	_____
❑	Mastering Stress	$ 9.95*	X _____	_____

* Purchase any four (4) tapes and get the fifth tape FREE!

TOTAL: _____

S&H: **$3.50**

AMOUNT ENCLOSED: _____

❑ Check/Cash   ❑ Visa/MasterCard   ❑ Amercian Express

Card # _____ Exp. _____

Signature _____ Date _____

Name _____

Address _____

City _____ State _____ Zip _____

Phone number (____) _____ — _____

To order simply tear out the order form and mail it to
The Optimal Performance Institute
520 S. Murphy Ave. Ste. 256, Sunnyvale, CA 94086
or call **1-800-607-0369**
or visit our website at **www.LivingLean.org**

Order Form

Please send me the following products & programs:

		Price	Quantity	TOTAL
❏	**PowerWalking!** System	$ 15.00	X _____	_____
❏	You will **Stop Smoking Now!**	$ 19.95	X _____	_____
❏	Nutra Trim	$ 11.95	X _____	_____
❏	Nutra Source 100	$ 23.95	X _____	_____
❏	**Living Lean!** Journal	$ 9.95	X _____	_____

Additional audiocassettes by John Farley:

		Price	Quantity	TOTAL
❏	Super Nutrition I	$ 9.95*	X _____	_____
❏	Super Nutrition II	$ 9.95*	X _____	_____
❏	Reverse Aging I	$ 9.95*	X _____	_____
❏	Reverse Aging II	$ 9.95*	X _____	_____
❏	Mastering Stress	$ 9.95*	X _____	_____

* Purchase any four (4) tapes and get the fifth tape FREE!

TOTAL: _____

S&H: **$3.50**

AMOUNT ENCLOSED: _____

❏ Check/Cash   ❏ Visa/MasterCard   ❏ Amercian Express

Card # _____ Exp. _____

Signature _____ Date _____

Name _____

Address _____

City _____ State _____ Zip _____

Phone number (____) _____ — _____

To order simply tear out the order form and mail it to
The Optimal Performance Institute
520 S. Murphy Ave. Ste. 256, Sunnyvale, CA 94086
or call **1-800-607-0369**
or visit our website at **www.LivingLean.org**